HONORING HOLISTIC HEALTH HABITS

Down to Dealing with Deadly Diets

HONORING HOLISTIC HEALTH HABITS

Down to Dealing with Deadly Diets

TOM TAYLOR

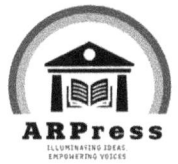

Copyright © 2024 by Tom Taylor

All rights reserved. No part of this publication may be reproduced, distributed, or transmitted in any form or by any means, including photocopying, recording, or other electronic or mechanical methods, without the prior written permission of the copyright owner and the publisher, except in the case of brief quotations embodied in critical reviews and certain other noncommercial uses permitted by copyright law. For permission requests, write to the publisher, addressed "Attention: Permissions Coordinator," at the address below.

ARPress
45 Dan Road Suite 5
Canton MA 02021
Hotline: 1(888) 821-0229
Fax: 1(508) 545-7580

Ordering Information:
Quantity sales. Special discounts are available on quantity purchases by corporations, associations, and others. For details, contact the publisher at the address above.

Printed in the United States of America.

ISBN-13: Paperback 979-8-89389-438-7
          eBook   979-8-89389-439-4

Library of Congress Control Number: 2024917385

The Alliterations: Four Books on Healthy Living

Overcoming Obesity
Working with Weight
Lifestyle and Longevity
Staying Alive: Down to Dealing with Deadly Diets

Tom Taylor, MD

Table of Contents

Preface i
Introduction iii

Part 1 : Avoiding Early Death by Maintaining Good Health Care

Chapter 1: The Heart. 1
Chapter 2 : Hypertension. 7
Chapter 3 : Arteriosclerosis and Stroke Arteriosclerosis 9
Chapter 4 : Prediabetes, Diabetes, and Syndrome X 12
Chapter 5 : Cancer. 19
Chapter 6 : Types of Cancer, Osteoarthritis, and Joint Disease . . 21
Chapter 7 : Obesity. 27
Chapter 8 : Obesity and Covid-19 35
Chapter 9 : Obesity and Life Expectancy 41
Chapter 10 : Reasons for Obesity. 44
Chapter 11 : The Effect That Technology Has Had on Lifestyle . 48
Chapter 12 : Psychological Factors 50
Chapter 13 : Alzheimer's Disease 53
Chapter 14 : Memory and the Effects of Diet. 60
Chapter 15 : Vaccination 63
Chapter 16 : Smoking 66
Chapter 17 : Non-alcoholic Fatty Disease of the Liver. 68

Chapter 18 : Illegal Drugs 69
Chapter 19 : Inflammatory Age. 71
Chapter 20 : Exercise. 74
Chapter 21: Sleep. 78
Chapter 22 : Further Psychological Factors 82

Part 2

Chapter 23 : How to Modify a Poor Diet. 89
Chapter 24 : Nutrition and Metabolism 95
Chapter 25 : Vegan and Vegetarian Diets 102
Chapter 26 : Dietary Methods for Reducing Weight 107
Chapter 27 : An Exciting New Development That Could Potentially Change the Playing Field 124
Chapter 28 : Conclusions: How Do I Stay Healthy? 126
Chapter 29 : Established Diagnostic Eating Disorders 134
Chapter 30 : In Conclusion 140

PREFACE

This book discusses in a comprehensive manner for the public the causes of the major killers in today's society and how these risks can be markedly reduced by lifestyle modification. Heart disease, stroke, obesity, diabetes, cancer, vascular disease, hypertension, and Alzheimer's disease are all primarily due to eating an unhealthy diet. These diseases have all dramatically increased over the last century as a result of the dietary changes that have taken place.

The nature of these diseases and the dietary impact underlying them is described along with the changes necessary to avoid and overcome them in an easy way. The issues underlying energy intake and expenditure, toxicity, and the dangers of the modern diet are emphasized. Present day diets contain unhealthy fats and toxic proteins, and they are loaded with excess carbohydrates, the latter being the major cause of weight gain and diabetes. Taken in the wrong amounts, these are all killers, which are now for the first time in centuries producing a reduction in life expectancy. How current dietary habits can be simply changed to prevent these diseases and increase longevity are discussed along with other preventative measures.

The primary quantitative eating disorders anorexia nervosa and bulimia, which are dramatically increasing particularly in the younger population, are also described.

Chapter 27 describes an exciting new development that could potentially change the playing field. A scientifically proven drug is now available to the obese majority, those in the highest risk group, to help reverse their deadly disorders.

The author has been a surgical gastroenterologist, a bariatric surgeon, and a professor of surgery in the Michael E. DeBakey Department of Surgery at Baylor College of Medicine. He has extensive experience of all aspects of his specialty and has had a particular interest in obesity and nutrition, having performed over 1000 gastric bypass procedures in the morbidly obese. The information presented in this book has been collected over many years from medical literature and clinical practice, and all aspects of it are considered to be scientifically accurate.

Introduction

There is a twenty-seven-year difference in life expectancy in different parts of the country.

What are the reasons for this? Clearly something could be done for improvement to level this out. Differing climates, occupations, or economic deprivation may play a part. It most probably comes down to diet, smoking, education, and social status. What are the major killers, what causes them, and how can they be avoided?

In this book I have concentrated on the major causes of early death and the investigation as to how these can be avoided. Is there something that they all have in common? The answer is that there is, and this is fundamentally down to diet.

Major changes in killing diseases have occurred over the last century and lifestyle has fundamentally changed to produce these. The average life expectation in 1900 was forty-two years, and presently it is in the high seventies, but now for the first time in over 100 years life expectation has begun to decline. How has lifestyle changed to produce these present-day killing diseases and increased their prevalence? The killing diseases today are heart disease hypertension, diabetes, stroke, cancer, infections, dementia, and pandemics. The major underlying factor for all of these is that they are eating disorders relating to modern diets. Mental illness, caused by stress, can also be related to eating disorders, and there are fundamental disorders of eating that can be fatal like anorexia nervosa and bulimia.

These diseases are potentially preventable, not only with dietary modification but in combination with exercise, sleeping correctly, and avoiding unnecessary stress. The issues are long-term, in fact lifelong, and can lead to early deaths in the thirties, forties, or even before. Let us look at the changes that have occurred and explain their role in present-day early death.

In 1948, the World Health Organization (WHO) defined health with a phrase that modern authorities still apply. "Health is a state of complete physical, mental and social well-being and not merely the absence of disease or infirmity." The word health therefore refers to a state of complete emotional well-being. Healthcare and health maintenance advice depends on helping people to maintain an optimal state of health within their own limitations and perhaps the multiple conditions and constraints to which they are subject.

According to the Center for Disease Control (CDC) healthcare costs in the United States are three and a half trillion dollars per year. Despite this, people in this country have a lower life expectancy than those in most other developed countries. This is due to a number of factors, importantly the structure and availability of healthcare, its costs, the national diet, and lifestyle choices.

A variety of definitions have been used over the years. Health can be promoted by encouraging activities such as regular physical exercise and adequate sleep and by avoiding smoking or excessive stress. Factors influencing health are due to individual choices, such as partaking in high-risk behaviors. Genetic factors may also be involved. The interpretation of the meaning of health has evolved over time. Early definitions related to the body's ability to function, which could be impaired by repeated diseases, such as infections, and this still applies but to different ones. Maintaining health requires the ability to deal with physical, biological, psychological and social stresses. The quoted 1948 WHO definition reported a departure from former ideas or definitions linking healthcare to well-being, but the factors herein are still of the utmost relevance today.

Over the last half of the twentieth century, life expectancy in Western countries improved substantially. Scientific advances in medicine have improved exponentially, and continue to do so, but there have also been setbacks. In 1950 there was no heart surgery, no tissue transplantation, no joint surgery, no intensive care units, only two simple antibiotics, virtually no chemotherapy, and few vaccines. Since the 1980s extension of life expectancy in the United States diverged to become ahead of that in other countries, but has now begun to decrease and the downward turn has continued in recent years. The reasons for this are discussed and are preventable.

PART 1

AVOIDING EARLY DEATH BY MAINTAINING GOOD HEALTH CARE

Chapter 1
The Heart

The twelve major causes of death today in Western countries are heart disease, cancer, accidents, chronic lower respiratory disease, stroke, Alzheimer's disease, diabetes, influenza and pneumonia, kidney disease, suicide, septicemia, and liver disease. Now additionally we have the problem of the Covid-19 pandemic, which is far from over and continues to present new and increasing scientific problems day by day. Heart disease and cancer are responsible for 46 percent of all deaths, the addition of chronic respiratory disease brings the figure to over 50 percent, and much can be done to maintain good health and avoid many of the deaths from these three causes. These twelve major causes account for 75 percent of all deaths.

Heart disease in the United States accounts for 650,000 deaths (23.1 percent). Those at higher risk are men, smokers, the obese, those with a family history, and those of increasing age. One person dies every thirty-seven seconds from heart disease in the United States, making it the major cause of death, and these numbers are increasing. It is estimated that by 2030, one million people in the US could die each year from heart disease. The major causes of heart disease are coronary artery disease, cardiac failure, heart arrhythmias, congenital defects and myocarditis.

The heart is an amazingly efficient pump that contracts at a rate of approximately seventy beats per minute for our whole lives. If we live to be eighty years or more, that's virtually three billion beats in a lifetime, which is extraordinary. The rate of contraction can vary from forty to two hundred or even more, but if it stops, death, initially due to lack of oxygen supply to the brain, occurs within two minutes. The heart has four chambers, two on the right and two on the left. The right side of the heart receives oxygen depleted blood from the veins throughout the whole body. The oxygen has been extracted by all of the tissues and organs, which is fundamentally essential for maintenance of their health and function. Blood that drains into the right side of the heart is expelled under a pressure of about 35 mm Hg from the right ventricle into the lungs where it is fully oxygenated and carbon dioxide is eliminated. The oxygenated blood then enters the left side of the heart, initially the left atrium, where it is expelled under low pressure into the relaxed left ventricle through the mitral valve. The strong, thick-walled left ventricle then contracts closing the mitral valve and pumping the oxygenated blood under high pressure through the arteries to the whole of the rest of the body, particularly the brain, the kidneys, and the liver and through every living piece of tissue, all of which require oxygen for their viability. The oxygen is extracted as the blood flows through these tissues and the deoxygenated blood enters the veins, which collect the blood under low pressure and return them to the right side of the heart. The height of the pressure generated by the left ventricle is normally about 120 mm Hg but this can increase to pressures in excess of 200 mm Hg in extreme cases of hypertension where this pressure damages not only the heart but the kidneys and other organs, frequently leading to stroke. Not only oxygen but all other important nutrients absorbed through the intestines are pumped to all of the body tissues to which it is essential for the maintenance of adequate nutrition.

Of the four chambers, the left and right atrium are the smaller, thinner-walled chambers that pump blood through the tricuspid and mitral valves into the relaxed ventricles. The chambers of the heart are connected by an electrical wiring system that controls the synchronizing of the contraction of the chambers and controls the frequency of heartbeats in accordance with the requirements of the body. Strenuous exercise, like running, can require more than a doubling of the resting heart rates transmitted through these electrical stimuli.

The heart receives its own blood supply, which is crucial to its function, through the coronary arteries. There are two main coronary arteries: the right and the left that have branches, the right circumflex and the left descending coronary arteries. These vessels run along the surface of the heart and supply oxygen-rich blood to the cardiac muscle. The heart lies in the central chest in a thin protective sac called the pericardium.

The heart beats about 100,000 times a day pumping blood around all of the tissues. The blood volume is about eight pints. Deoxygenated blood, as stated, is pumped into the lungs that saturate it with oxygen and exhale carbon dioxide. The muscular tissue of the heart that causes contraction is referred to as the myocardium, and there is an inner lining throughout all of the chambers called the endocardium.

Each heartbeat has two components. Diastole is a period of relaxation when the ventricles fill with blood and systole is a period of muscular contraction of the ventricles and relaxation and filling of the atria. The pulse is created by contraction of the left ventricle pushing blood through the arterial system. The four heart valves open to allow blood to pass forward through the system and close to prevent any backflow.

Heart Disease

Heart disease remains the major killer in Western society. It describes a number of conditions, chiefly coronary artery disease, heart failure, and heart rhythm problems, known as arrhythmias, which can cause sudden death. Congenital heart lesions are a variable array of disorders of the structure of the heart, its vessels, or its valves. Heart valve disease can develop later in life. There are primary diseases that develop in heart muscle; the heart is prone to either viral or bacterial infections, and the pericardium surrounding the heart can be diseased as a result of a variety of conditions. Heart failure can develop from any of the above disorders.

Coronary artery disease was rare in the 1800s but with the turn of that century there was a rapid and progressive increase throughout the 1900s up to the year 2000, after which as a result of better prevention and treatment there has been a fall from 900,000 deaths per year to 700,000 in 2010. After this time, it began to increase again reaching over 800,000 deaths per year—this is over 25 percent of all deaths. Last year when it was at its height, Covid-19 accounted for 10.2 percent of deaths; worldwide, it has now killed over five million people.

Coronary artery disease develops when streaks of cholesterol are deposited on the inner lining of the coronary vessels. This occurs as a result of high blood levels of cholesterol and the deposits begin to develop at points where the blood vessels branch and divide. These are sites at which turbulence occurs in the blood flow and the turbulence accelerates the deposition of cholesterol. With increasing periods of time, the cholesterol streaks become confluent around the vessels. They also harden forming plaques. An acute event can then occur when a blood clot or thrombus attaches itself to the atheromatous plaque and completely occludes the coronary artery. This is the condition of coronary thrombosis or myocardial infarction, which kills the cardiac muscle supplied by the occluded artery.

The major factor in causing the increase in cardiac deaths, which are definitely dietary in causation, is the rise in low-density lipoprotein cholesterol, which is bad cholesterol. This is a modifiable risk factor whose relationship with cardiovascular disease has been well-established, and lowering the low density lipoprotein cholesterol reduces the risk of severe cardiac events. Several trials have shown that lowering low density lipoprotein cholesterol can reduce cardiac-related mortality by at least 30 percent, and for every 14 mg/dL of LDL reduction patients experience a 22 percent reduction of major adverse cardiac events, these figures being based upon clinical trials that included 170,000 participants with a follow-up of four to eight years. The longer patients have persistently elevated LDL cholesterol the earlier they are at risk of myocardial infarction; this increases with time in an exponential manner. It has been shown that up to 80 percent of patients with high LDL cholesterol levels are not reaching the recommended target of less than 70 mg/dL in their blood. The correct diet will reduce LDL cholesterol more than exercise and by adhering to it many can achieve favorable levels, though some require supplemental statin therapy, and new cholesterol-lowering drugs given by intravascular injection are showing dramatic reductions in the longer term. Those taking statins may experience intolerable side effects such as muscular pain and diseases, and sometimes even with statins recorded levels cannot be reduced to an adequate level and alternative treatments are required, which places greater emphasis on diet. There are some socioeconomic problems related to healthcare insurance and decline in health from Covid-19 infection has a deleterious effect. Lack of knowledge and patient education is another factor, so with other strategies available the patient should be tested regularly, they should know their numbers and the goals to achieve through the right sort of diet.

To prevent the narrowing of coronary arteries by cholesterol or thrombus, it is strongly advisable to eat correctly throughout life. First and foremost, it is essential to maintain a healthy weight. This is achieved by eating the right foods and taking moderate physical exercise, which includes walking, at least thirty minutes a day, though this may be divided into smaller walks. Food intake needs to decrease.

A diet rich in vegetables, and to a lesser extent fruit, reduces the risk of heart disease. The whole vegetable or fruit should be eaten as this contains fiber in the peel, which helps with vitamin and mineral intake while being low in calories. Potatoes are excluded from the above. Green or deeply colored vegetables are best. Brown rice is healthier than white; it is encased in a whole grain, which is good for heart health, whereas white rice is largely pure carbohydrate. Protein is contained in plants like legumes, including soybeans, tofu, lentils, chickpeas, split peas, and flax seed. Plant-based proteins are healthier than meat alternatives that may be ultra-processed and contain added sugar, saturated fat, salt stabilizers, and preservatives of fat. A regular intake of fish and seafood is recommended as they contain omega-3 fatty acids. Baked fish is healthier than fried fish. Skimmed milk and low-fat dairy products can be taken in moderation. White meat poultry, chicken, and turkey are high in protein and low in fat. Red meats like steak, bacon, sausage, hot dogs, and salami are high in fat, salt, and LDL cholesterol and should be avoided. Plant oils such as olive, canola, sunflower, soybean, corn, safflower, sunflower, and flaxseed oil are healthy. Coconut oil, butter, lard, and trans fats are unhealthy. Processed foods contain added sugar, salt, and fats or other preservatives and should be avoided, so home-cooked vegetables and boiled fish are always preferred. Examples of highly processed foods are store purchased cakes, cookies, pizzas, and pies.

When preparing food at home, little or no salt should be added as salt has an effect on baroreceptors in the carotid arteries causing an elevation of blood pressure.

Minimize sugary drinks and foods. Added sugars like glucose, sucrose, honey, maple syrup, and concentrated fruit juice are associated with a high risk of type II diabetes. A can of Coke, for example, contains the equivalent of nine teaspoons of sugar. Alcohol consumption should be limited; however, there is conflicting evidence about moderate alcohol intake as red wine may be protective to the heart though the topic is controversial.

A diabetes drug could transform the treatment of heart failure and cut deaths by more than one fifth, doctors have recently revealed. Half of heart failure patients have reduced ejection fraction, where the heart is unable to pump blood around the body due to a mechanical issue. Half have preserved ejection fraction, where the heart pumps blood well but cannot provide oxygen to all parts of the body. It has recently been shown that drugs named SGLT2 inhibitors, the semaglutides, which are used to treat diabetes, could aid patients with reduced ejection fraction. These medications can improve the outcomes for people in heart failure with low ejection fractions and they could revolutionize treatment offered to heart failure patients.

CHAPTER 2
HYPERTENSION

Almost 50 percent of adults in the United States have hypertension or high blood pressure. This is an important underlying feature to the development of coronary artery disease, heart failure, cardiac arrhythmias, and stroke. Other side effects are aneurysm, kidney disease, and dementia.

High blood pressure occurs because the heart has to use increased force to overcome the peripheral resistance created by hardening of the arteries as a result of arteriosclerosis. The major factor in damaging the arteries and causing hypertension is again an unhealthy diet. Other predisposing factors are family history, increasing age, and lack of exercise. Hypertension is sometimes referred to as the silent killer as it typically does not produce any signs or symptoms in affected individuals before it strikes, sometimes suddenly and fatally, with either a stroke or heart attack. The pressure increases slowly over the years but may produce headaches, shortness of breath, nosebleeds, and visual disturbance even leading to blindness.

You can measure your blood pressure easily and frequently by purchasing an inexpensive device that inflates around the upper arm and can accurately record systolic and diastolic blood pressure which should be below 140 and 90 mm Hg respectively.

Blood pressure can be controlled at very safe levels of the order of 120/80 by first concentrating once again on eating a healthy diet rich in vegetables and fruits, reducing red meat and animal fat and cutting down on salt. Maintaining a healthy weight is important and, again, smoking should be completely avoided. Try to reduce and manage stress and sleep well. There are a number of medications that are highly efficient in the control of blood pressure such as lisinopril, metoprolol, hydrochlorothiazide, and others. Moderate exercise should be part of your healthy living plan, which will help to control blood pressure. Again, the major cause and one which is remedial is diet.

Chapter 3
Arteriosclerosis and Stroke
Arteriosclerosis

Arteriosclerosis or hardening of the arteries is the fundamental problem that underlies all of the other major current killers, coronary artery disease, heart failure, stroke, diabetes, and dementia. It is basically caused by bad diet as are all of the other major killers. Close to one million people per year die in the United States of diseases caused by arteriosclerosis.

In early life the arteries throughout our bodies are smooth and elastic, lined by a smooth glistening lining called endothelium. Arteriosclerosis that today affects, to some extent, almost all adults begins by a buildup of streaks of cholesterol on the endothelium as described above in the coronary arteries. The streaks buildup and become confluent around the whole blood vessel, they develop particularly in relation to points at which blood vessels branch. High levels of bad LDL cholesterol in the bloodstream taken in the diet accelerate this process. The cholesterol lining becomes hardened and irregular and is then referred to as plaque. Certain vessels are particularly predisposed to the buildup mainly those close to junctions and branches. These, in addition to the coronary arteries, are the carotid arteries in the neck, which are the major source of blood supply to the brain and whose occlusion causes stroke; the femoral vessels in the legs, which when blocked can lead to gangrene and amputation; and the main blood vessel in the body, the abdominal aorta. The irregular buildup of plaque within these vessels narrows the arteries and causes turbulent flow that also occurs in relation to arterial branches, and blood clots form on these causing thrombosis that can be suddenly fatal, as pointed out in the coronary arteries, and it can also occur in the major arteries to the brain or lower limbs. Sudden occlusion of the carotid arteries in the neck is the major cause of stroke. Occlusion of the femoral artery in the leg leads to gangrene necessitating amputation often above the knee. So arteriosclerosis is the major killer underlying every disease that accounts for the main causes of death in Western countries.

Stroke

A stroke occurs as a result of the blood supply to an essential part of the brain being suddenly blocked or from hemorrhage into the brain. Loss of oxygen to the brain rapidly, within a couple of minutes, leads to damage to the part of the brain affected and this area dies, resulting in the loss of function to the parts of the body that this part of the brain controls. There are four main arteries to the brain, the largest being the right and left carotid arteries that run up the side of the neck to enter the brain through a hole in the base of the skull. The other two arteries are the vertebral arteries that run along the right and left side of the vertebrae in the neck to enter the skull. The commonest cause of stroke is related to arteriosclerosis of the carotid artery close to the point where it divides into two branches, internal and external, close to the base of the skull. This produces narrowing of the vessel that ultimately undergoes thrombosis and blockage of blood supply to an essential part of the brain. These types of strokes are referred to as ischemic strokes.

The other type of stroke that occurs when a blood vessel in the brain bursts and leaks into the brain is called a hemorrhagic stroke. This also leads to a cutoff to the supply of blood to the adjacent part of the brain, which is damaged by the accumulating blood.

Again, the causes are arteriosclerosis leading to narrowing of the arteries and sometimes to spontaneous rupture of a vessel are bad diet and high cholesterol levels. Once again, the major cause is hypertension.

A rare type of stroke, again due to arteriosclerosis, occurs when a clot forms in another part of the body and travels through the bloodstream to block an artery inside the brain. The commonest origins of these clots is in the atrium of the heart and the chest or upper neck. This type of stroke is described as a cerebral embolism. The latter type of strokes have the same underlying causes as other strokes, chiefly bad diet, hypertension, and smoking, but atrial fibrillation, an abnormality of cardiac contraction, is also a common cause of cerebral embolism.

Over 200,000 cases of stroke occur each year in the United States, and 87 percent of these are ischemic. There are often heralding signs like the development of weakness of limbs or a speech problem. The major risk factors include a bad diet, diabetes, heart disease, hypertension, obesity, sedentary lifestyle high blood cholesterol levels, and family history. There are some racial differences as well; for example, African Americans run a higher risk.

These risk factors, which are common to all the major killers, can be controlled with healthy lifestyle changes. Eating a healthy diet is, again, the basic necessity along with increasing exercise, controlling blood pressure and, of course. not smoking.

CHAPTER 4
PREDIABETES, DIABETES, AND SYNDROME X

PREDIABETES

About sixty million people in the United States have prediabetes. Prediabetes is not only the forerunner of diabetes itself, but that of all of the major killers described. Prediabetes is diagnosed when the fasting blood glucose is between 100 and 125 mg/dl on more than one occasion. Diabetes is diagnosed when the fasting blood glucose is 126 mg/dL or greater on more than one occasion. Prediabetes is also diagnosed when the blood glucose two hours after eating seventy-five grams of glucose is between 140 and 200 mg/dL. Despite its massive prevalence the term prediabetes has not been around long. In fact, it was first used in 2002 when it was introduced by the American Diabetes Association. Studies have shown that most people with prediabetes will ultimately go on within the next ten years to develop diabetes itself unless they change their diet and exercise profile. Having a diagnosis of prediabetes puts a person at a 50 percent greater risk of a heart attack or stroke. Factors predisposing to prediabetes are obesity, hypertension, sedentary lifestyle, and high levels of triglyceride and cholesterol. It is also more common in certain ethnic groups particularly African Americans. Prediabetes is a forerunner of heart attacks, strokes, blindness, due to retinopathy, renal impairment, and Alzheimer's disease. The elderly are at the greatest risk of developing prediabetes or diabetes, about one third of people aged sixty-five or older have diabetes. A further 30 percent have prediabetes. About a third of elderly patients have neither of these conditions that form the basis upon which all the other major killers accrue. Stress plays an important role in prediabetes.

Prediabetes occurs principally as a result of any of the following factors: eating a little more food each day than you need for your daily activities resulting in increased weight, drinking sugary sodas instead of water, eating foods high in saturated fats and trans fatty acids, drinking too much alcohol, and taking little exercise.

The reason why there has been such a massive increase of prediabetes and diabetes relates to the evolution of our food supply. Humans began as hunter gatherers and continued to obtain their food in that way for thousands of years. They hunted for meat in the forests, ate berries from the trees, picked grasses, and found wild fruit. About 10,000 years ago communities gathered together and began to stabilize, and agriculture began with the planting of crops. It was then possible to store some of these crops throughout the winter and also to keep animals in fields where they could provide protein. With the industrial revolution cities grew at a tremendous pace and food became available firstly in shops, and later in the ubiquitous supermarket. Improved agriculture led to the production of large amounts of corn that was fed to cattle, but also provided a huge source of cheap calories that were incorporated into new kinds of food products, such as breakfast cereal. These refined carbohydrates were also added to sodas and used as sweeteners and preservatives for so many foods that could be maintained in an edible state for long periods of time. The refined carbohydrates in supermarket foods is converted into fat in the liver and provides an easy source of multiple calories. In addition, the refined carbohydrates boost blood glucose stimulating insulin production and forming a basis for prediabetes. As carbohydrates are refined all the good nutrients are removed as the grain has been stripped away. It is the increased consumption of refined carbohydrates that has formed the basis for the development of prediabetes and ultimately all of the major killers.

Diabetes

There are two types of diabetes type I and type II. Type I diabetes is much less common and is unrelated to type ll. In Type I there is a lack of functional insulin secreting cells in the pancreas, which prevents insulin from breaking down glucose, so it builds up in the bloodstream. This occurs frequently in young people and is often familial.

Type II diabetes mellitus is also a disease of the pancreas, which produces the hormone, insulin, that helps regulate blood sugar levels. More than forty million Americans now have diabetes according to the Centers for Disease Control and Prevention (CDC), which is approximately 10 percent of the population. The disease can be reversed and respond if associated with the right sort of lifestyle changes. The Surgeon General's reports have estimated the costs of obesity in the United States to be $150 billion per year. One half of this money is spent on treating the complications of diabetes or other conditions produced by diabetes such as heart attacks, stroke, kidney failure, and blindness. We hear so much of the detrimental effects of smoking and drinking, but diabetes outranks both of these and has markedly deteriorating effects on health. Of the two types of diabetes, type II is by far and away the most common and can be reversed in a large proportion who undergo obesity surgery. Obesity surgery commonly cures not only diabetes but reduces the associated risks.

Insulin production and utilization is the key to diabetes that allows sugar to enter the cell and provide energy. When the lock is faulty, sugars cannot enter the cells, and they build up in the bloodstream where they cause damage. Carrying excess fat adds to the difficulty that insulin has in doing its job. If the sugar cannot enter the cells, the pancreas goes on pumping out more and more insulin in response to the high blood sugar. Ultimately the insulin may overshoot the mark and produce a rapid falling of blood sugar, which can cause powerful appetite stimulation. Diabetics whose blood sugar is poorly controlled are continuously pouring out excess insulin to which they become increasingly resistant. Insulin resistance is the fundamental problem in the long term associated with type II diabetes. The high levels of blood sugar damage other organs in particular the eye and the kidney, leading to blindness and renal failure. Extremes of blood sugar concentrations, both low and high, may lead to coma, which is life-threatening. Diabetics also develop accelerated arteriosclerosis with the increased risk of all the other major killers.

The following factors increase the risk of developing diabetes: obesity, a family history of diabetes, use of certain medications, injury to the pancreas, a predisposition to an autoimmune disease like rheumatoid arthritis, high blood pressure, heavy alcohol use, smoking, and advanced age.

With regard to risk factors for diabetes the more fatty tissue you have in your body the more resistant your cells become to insulin. The less active you are, the greater your risk. Physical activity helps you to control your weight, uses up glucose as energy and makes your cells more sensitive to insulin. Having a family history of diabetes is a risk factor; certain ethnic groups including African and Asian American people are at higher risk. The disease gets more common with increasing age when the amount of exercise is reduced and people lose muscle mass, but type II diabetes is also increasing in children and adolescents where it is increasingly being observed.

The type of diabetes in children is changing. It used to be that they got the more aggressive, often inherited Type 1 diabetes. Now, in addition, they are developing type II diabetes at a massive rate. Over a ten-year period, there has been a staggering 500 percent increase in type II diabetes in children, and these children are invariably obese. The prevalence of type II diabetes in Americans has escalated exponentially so that now more than twenty states have a prevalence of obesity greater than 25 percent of the population.

As it has been pointed out, for many thousands of years ancient man ate unrefined carbohydrates as part of the hunter-gatherer type of diet. With these diets, the pancreas was stimulated to a much lesser extent than with current diets. Until 200 years ago, humans ate less than one pound of refined sugar per year. Now, 150 pounds are eaten each year. Sugar manufacturers, producers, and the packaged food industry have paved the way to the current situation. However, cynical as it might sound, the sugar manufacturers have contributed to the deaths of more Americans than all wars combined.

We eat carbohydrates in the form of simple sugars and starches, all carbohydrates are eventually broken down to the simple sugar glucose. Glucose maintains the blood sugar at a steady level in the non-diabetic. Small amounts, about 600 grams, are stored in the liver and to a lesser extent in muscle, any remaining glucose is converted into and stored as fat. Glucose comes from two major sources: food and your liver. Sugar is absorbed into the bloodstream where it enters the cells with the help of insulin. The liver stores and also makes glucose. When glucose levels are low, such as after a period of fasting, the liver breaks down stored glycogen, a complex series of glucose molecules, into glucose to keep your glucose level within the normal range. Normal people secrete about twenty-five to thirty units of insulin per day. Insulin sweeps glucose into the cells where it is stored. Insulin prevents the level of glucose in the blood from rising. Conversely glucagon, another hormone, in the fasting state, prevents the blood sugar from falling too low. Too much insulin can produce dangerously low levels of blood sugar.

Glucagon is a second important hormone in the pancreas and acts, in many ways, in an opposite way to insulin. Glucagon is released by a protein stimulus, not glucose. Glucagon promotes the mobilization of previously stored fat, so you burn body fat in response to this hormone rather than store it in response to insulin. Carbohydrate rich meals suppress glucagon secretion. The continued excessive stimulus to insulin production created by a high carbohydrate diet ultimately produces insulin resistance, which is a diminished effect of insulin in response to more sugar.

Excessive glucose intake over time, therefore, produces insulin resistance. There is then a decreased responsiveness to insulin wherein fat cells, liver cells, and muscle cells become insensitive to insulin and blood glucose concentrations rise. Insulin resistance is a major and the most dangerous factor in the development of obesity. The higher levels of circulating insulin cause the body to store as much fat as is possible. Insulin resistance is also the fundamental problem underlying many of the other major killers. Reducing the intake of sugar will lower the peak insulin levels and will ultimately reduce insulin resistance. The precise reasons why insulin resistance occurs are not fully understood, but it is reversible. Insulin resistance can run in families and is made worse by unhealthy lifestyle habits. These habits are, lack of exercise, poor diet and both nutritional deficiencies and excesses of substance abuse, smoking and drinking.

The symptoms of diabetes vary depending upon the degree of elevation of the blood glucose. Those with prediabetes or early diabetes may sometimes have no symptoms as the disease becomes established and the blood glucose becomes persistently elevated. In type II diabetes, the symptoms are increased thirst, frequent urination, extreme hunger, unexplained weight loss, fatigue, irritability, blurred vision, slow healing sores, and frequent infection of the skin or vagina.

The complications of diabetes are the development of all of the other major causes of early death discussed herein. Diabetes dramatically increases the risk of coronary artery disease, heart failure, hypertension, and stroke. Once again, it is down to arteriosclerosis due to abnormal diet. Other problems that develop in the diabetic patient are nerve damage, kidney damage, retinopathy, or damage to the eye, all of which are due to damage to the blood vessels supplying these organs as a result of arteriosclerosis. Alzheimer's disease and depression also occur with increased incidence in the diabetic.

Prevention of diabetes again comes down to lifestyle changes first and foremost eating a healthy diet with foods lower in sugar, fat, and overall calories, just as in arteriosclerosis and all of the other major killers discussed. Once again, focus on vegetables, fruit, and whole grains. Increased physical activity and the loss of excess weight are also important. Details of the dietary changes common to all of these diseases are discussed in later chapters.

Halting the development of diabetes can be achieved by observing the following parameters.

1. Cut down on the total amount of food you eat.
2. Increase exercise and avoid sitting in front of the television or computer for the day.
3. Avoid sugary drinks, as one can of Coke contains nine teaspoons of sugar.
4. Avoid foods containing trans fatty acids.
5. Reduce salt intake.

6. Keep alcohol intake within the normal parameters outlined.
7. If needed take statins in order to reduce your cholesterol and triglycerides addressed by your doctor.

Syndrome X

Obesity is more than a cosmetic problem. It is the direct cause of the whole process of medical problems discussed herein that are the biggest killers of American citizens today. The three most important problems associated with the obese state are high blood pressure, high blood cholesterol concentrations, and diabetes mellitus. This trio is often referred to as syndrome X. Seventy million Americans suffer from syndrome X, the components of which are linked by sugar intolerance to insulin resistance. The collection of problems now represents the number one public health initiative facing Western society. Our current lifestyle and behavior is largely responsible for this syndrome, the sedentary lifestyle watching television, sitting in front of computers, and driving everywhere. As stated, over the past century technological developments have almost completely removed physical exercise from day-to-day lives. In association with diet, this lifestyle sets the scene for the major killers. The syndrome now affects not only the elderly or the middle aged; it is also having a major effect on children and teenagers.

Chapter 5
Cancer

Cancer is a group of diseases in which previously normal cells in the body undergo change and grow uncontrollably, ultimately spreading to other parts of the body. Cancer can arise in almost any group of cells in the body that continue to duplicate and invade other cells and other organs in the body. The body consists of trillions of cells that in the developmental process differ and form all of the major organs. These are stem cells that continue to grow and multiply throughout life with new cells replacing replete cells. If a mutation in the cellular structure occurs, these new cells become abnormal and continue to grow in this abnormal form, out of basic control. The growth of the cells can cause masses or lumps in the body that invade or obstruct other organs, or spread through the lymphatics or bloodstream to invade other organs. These areas of spread are referred to as metastases. Many cancers form solid tumors, but cancers of the bloodstream, the leukemias, destroy the blood-producing bone marrow and prevent the development of normal red and white blood cells.

A group of tumors referred to as benign do not spread or invade adjacent tissues but they can grow to a large size and compress or damage adjacent structures such as the brain. Cancerous changes in cells are caused by changes in the genes that control normal cellular function. These changes occur as cells incorrectly divide and the abnormal genes proliferate in the cancerous tissue. The damage to genes occurs as a result of exposure to harmful substances, such as those in unhealthy foods and in tobacco. As the cancer grows further, genetic changes tend to occur in the cells. Abnormal genetic changes are common, but most are destroyed by the body and fail to proliferate. Some, however, are resistant to this protective mechanism. Oncogenes, genes that can cause normal cells to develop into tumor cells, are more aggressive and are the basis of many cancers. Tumor suppressor genes tend to prevent the development of an aggressive malignant process. Most people who die of cancer do so because of the damaging effects of the metastases in different parts of the body. The commonest forms of cancer and the major killers are adenocarcinomas that occur in the breast, colon, stomach, prostate, uterus, and ovary. Lung cancer, which is of a different cell type, is in the majority of cases related to smoking. The other cancers share the same basic developmental problems as occur with all the other major killers described in this book.

Breast, colon, uterus, and ovarian cancers occur with increasing incidence as a result of the same dietary indiscretions that lead to the other major killers and, while not reversible, their incidence can be reduced by employing the same dietary guidelines as are described in the latter part of this book. They all share the same common factors in their development.

Chapter 6
Types of Cancer, Osteoarthritis, and Joint Disease

Lung Cancer

Lung cancer remains the commonest form of malignant disease and is different in its etiology than the other major solid tumors described herein. This is not a disease related to diet but is directly related to smoking. Smoking should be absolutely banned from your life as it is the worst thing you can do. Many legal measures have been introduced in recent years to prevent smoking in bars, restaurants, public places, and even in some areas in the streets. Governments have increased smoking deterrence by increasing the price of cigarettes and placing figurative warnings on the packets. New Zealand has now completely banned cigarettes from the country.

Lung carcinomas derive from transformed malignant cells that originate as epithelial or skin-like cells from the tissues derived from this type of cells. There are other types of lung cancer that are rare. These are sarcomas, generated by the malignant transformation of connective tissues, arising from nerve fat muscle and bone. In time the uncontrolled growth of cells spreads beyond the lung either by direct invasion of adjacent tissues, by spread through the lymphatic system, or by direct invasion of and spread through the bloodstream. This spread can occur to the brain, liver, bones or other tissues. There are two main types of carcinoma of the lung, small cell and nonsmall cell.

The main symptoms of lung cancer are dry cough, sometimes with the production of blood, breathlessness and chest pain.

At least 85 percent of lung cancers are due to long-term tobacco smoking, but about 10 percent occur in nonsmokers. These can be due to genetic factors, exposure to radiation or asbestos, and exposure to secondhand smoke, which has now largely been eliminated from public places.

Worldwide in 2020, lung cancer occurred in 2.2 million people and resulted in 1.8 million deaths, indicating its extremely high mortality. It is the most common cause of cancer-related deaths in men and the second most common in women, after breast cancer. Most cases occur beyond the age of sixty and increase annually with age thereafter. In the United States, the five-year survival rate is 20.5 percent, while in Japan it is as high as 41 percent.

Cigarette smoke contains over seventy known carcinogens. Passive smoking is due to the prolonged exposure in rooms filled with an atmosphere of smoke; sometimes you can't see across the room. Under these circumstances, the incidence of lung cancer increases by almost 25 percent compared with the nonexposed population.

Electronic cigarettes, cigars, pipe smoking, and tobacco chewing increase the risk, as probably does the smoking of marijuana. Radiation and asbestos exposure can also increase the risk. Outdoor air pollution from chemical factories and traffic exhaust fumes can also predispose us to cancer. Generally, these latter overall play a minor role.

COLON CANCER

There are approximately 150,000 cases of colon cancer in the United States per annum and 50,000 in the United Kingdom. This is an 8 percent incidence of all cancers. In the US, there are 53,000 deaths per year with a five-year survival rate of 65 percent. Both the incidence of the disease and the mortality have declined by about 20 percent in the last twenty years.

Risk factors for colon cancer include diet, obesity, lack of physical activity, and smoking. Dietary factors that increase the incidence include red meat consumption, processed meats, and possibly alcohol. People who have preexisting ulcerative colitis or Crohn's disease have a very definite increased incidence of the disease. Some genetic disorders can place people at higher risk, particularly adenomatous polyposis where the incidence of subsequent cancer is virtually 100 percent. Other genes can also play a part. Recent research has shown a link between sugar sweetened drinks and bowel cancer, and it found in adults, particularly women, drinking two or more sodas each day doubles the risk of bowel cancer before the age of fifty. Soft drinks, fruit flavored drinks, as well as sports and energy drinks all pose a significant threat the study showed.

Screening by checking for blood in the stools and carrying out a colonoscopic examination of the colon is recommended starting at the age of fifty. A polyp is a precancerous condition and if detected early at colonoscopy cancer can either be prevented or easily cured by removal of the polyp. The other important mode of prevention is adhering to the dietary recommendations described herein.

Breast Cancer

Breast cancer develops as a lump within the tissues of the breast. It is the most common cancer diagnosed in women in the United States. About 1 percent of breast cancers occur in males. The commonest presentation is that of a lump or thickening within the breast tissue that feels much firmer than the surrounding tissue. Sometimes it involves the overlying skin producing multiple small pits like those on the surface of an orange. Occasionally, if a tumor is large, it can alter the shape or appearance of the breast. Sometimes the nipple may become inverted. Most women present to their doctors having noticed a palpable lump within their breast tissue. The tumor usually slowly grows and ultimately spreads through the lymphatic system to lymph nodes under the arm. It may also enter the bloodstream and spread throughout the body particularly to bone. The tumor most often begins with cells in the milk-producing ducts but can sometimes occur in the lobules or larger fatty cells within the breast substance. Risk factors for breast cancer are dietary or genetic. About 5 to 10 percent of breast cancers are linked to gene mutations passed through generations of a family. Some families pass on an inherited mutated gene either BRCA1 or BRCA2, both of which massively increase the risk of breast and ovarian cancer. Risk factors for breast cancer are the female sex, increasing age, a personal history of breast conditions like the removal of benign lumps, a family history of breast cancer, or the presence of one of the above genes. Obesity is also a risk factor. Young girls beginning to menstruate before the age of twelve increases the risk, also going through the menopause at an older age is a risk factor. Women who have never been pregnant and those who have been on hormone therapy during the menopause also have an increased risk. It has been suggested that drinking alcohol is a risk factor, though there is not a lot of evidence about this. Again, dietary factors are important in the development of this disease.

It is important for women to carry out self-examination of their breasts and beyond the age of fifty undergo mammography, an X-ray test on the breast tissue. The duration of postmenopausal hormone therapy should be reduced, and it seems as though, as with the other major killers, regular exercise, amounting to thirty minutes on most days of the week, is a protective factor along with the latter two considerations, maintaining a healthy weight and eating a healthy diet. It has been shown that women who eat a Mediterranean diet supplemented with extra virgin oil and mixed nuts may have a reduced risk of breast cancer. The Mediterranean diet focuses mostly on plant-based foods such as fruits and vegetables, whole grains, legumes and nuts. Using olive oil rather than butter and fish instead of red meat is also protective. Estrogen blocking medications reduce the risk of cancer in women who are at high risk of the disease. Those with a very high risk may choose to have their breasts surgically removed and replaced by implants.

Prostate Cancer

Prostate cancer occurs as a result of the development of invasive cells within the substance of the prostate, which is a walnut-shaped structure sitting below the bladder. Prostate cancer is one of the most common types of cancer and is very prevalent in elderly males. The malignant cells within the prostate grow and invade other organs, particularly the bone. Some tumors are slowly progressive, others develop rapidly. The symptoms of prostate cancer are difficulty in passing urine, blood in the urine, weight loss, bone pain, and erectile dysfunction. Risk factors are increasing age, African American race, or family history. Obesity is another risk factor, and dietary factors are once again important in the development of this disease. These are the same dietary factors that relate to all of the other disorders discussed herein.

The best way to avoid the risk of prostate cancer is, to once again, eat a healthy diet with fruits and vegetables together with whole grains. As with many other diseases considered, exercise on a daily basis is an important factor as is maintaining a healthy or normal weight.

Ovarian Cancer

Ovarian cancer occurs as a result of the development of massive abnormal cells within the ovarian tissue. The ovary is the size of a walnut and two of them exist, one on either side of the uterus. Symptoms are late to develop but ultimately abdominal bloating or swelling may occur with weight loss and pelvic discomfort, urinary frequency, or a change in bowel habit may also develop. The causation of ovarian cancer is not fully understood, but once again dietary factors appear to be important. Other risk factors are increasing age, genetic factors, and a family history of ovarian cancer. Obesity is a risk factor, and ovarian cancer occurs more frequently in those who began menstruation at an early age or develop the menopause at a later age. Never having been pregnant is another risk factor.

Uterine Cancer

The uterus is a pear-shaped organ that lies in the center of the female pelvis and in which fetuses develop. The disease frequently presents with the vaginal bleeding or pelvic pain. The exact causes of uterine cancer are not fully understood, but again dietary factors appear to be important, hormonal factors also predispose. Obesity is also a risk factor as is hormone therapy.

Osteoarthritis and Joint Disease

Another rapidly increasing disease that predisposes to and underlies other causes of increasing mortality is degenerative joint disease or osteoarthritis, affecting mainly the hip and knee joints. Osteoarthritis is a wear and tear disease that destroys cartilage within the joints and erodes the underlying bone. The joints are lined by cartilage that forms a smooth, low friction layer over the bone, which articulates in the joint space. Once again, poor nutrition is a major underlying causative factor that is obesity created by bad nutrition. Obesity causes excess pressure within the hip and knee joints that increases friction within the joint spaces and wears away the cartilage. Eventually the bone itself in the joint becomes damaged producing severe pain and markedly restricted movement.

Obesity is the major risk factor here as well, as it markedly increases pressure in the joint space and restricts both movement in the joint and walking. The lack of mobility that this produces leads to a further progression of the disease and a further increase in weight.

Chapter 7
Obesity

Being overweight purely and simply means that the body is carrying too much fat. Eating many more calories than the body is burning up, whether these are carbohydrates or fat, results in fat being accumulated. By and large, the excess intake of carbohydrate is responsible, and this is converted into and stored throughout the body as fat. As excess fat is accumulated, it leads to the state of obesity.

If someone gains ten pounds in weight, that is the equivalent of a bucket full of fat being distributed mainly around the abdomen, the upper abdomen in males and the lower abdomen and pelvis in females. Some of this fat will also go to the thighs. The person is then carrying this bucket of fat everywhere they go, every time they move. Being overweight is now the major risk factor for reducing your life expectancy, killing even more than smoking as more people are continuing to become overweight and fewer are smoking. It is also the major risk factor associated with morbidity and mortality in the Covid 19 crisis.

Obesity is the basis of type II diabetes, hypertension, coronary artery disease, and stroke and further adds to risk a predisposition to cause death from Covid-19. The United States has the largest obesity problem in the world, and at the time of writing, has the highest mortality from Covid disease, approximately 500,000 deaths. In Europe, the United Kingdom is the most obese nation and has the highest death toll of all the European countries.

The word obesity refers to an excess of body fat. This is measured by having a body mass index of 28 kg/m2 or a weight 20 percent or more above the ideal body weight. About 100 million adults in the United States are obese by this definition. Of these some eight million have a body mass index of over 40 kg/m2, meaning that they suffer from severe or morbid obesity, the risks of which are life-threatening. This number has doubled in the last ten years and continues to rapidly increase.

The rates of obesity are rapidly increasing among Americans of all ages, ethnicities, and socioeconomic groups. Presently, they are highest among African Americans and Hispanics. One of the most alarming statistics is that one in five American children between the ages of six and eighteen years is now obese. In the last ten years over two million teenagers and young adults joined the ranks of the clinically obese. Americans spend fifty billion dollars per year on diets and weight reducing methods. The annual medical costs relating to obesity in the USA are approaching $100 billion per year. The average person in the United States consumes some 150 pounds of refined sugar per year, compared with one pound a century ago, and this excess sugar consumption is directly related to the obesity crisis. It is excess carbohydrate intake that is the major causative factor.

Obesity is more than a cosmetic problem. It is the direct cause of the major medical problems killing people today. The three most important problems associated with the obese state are high blood pressure, high blood cholesterol, and diabetes mellitus. This trio is the basis of all of the major killers outlined in this text apart from lung cancer, which is clearly a smoking-related disease. This collection of problems now presents the number one public health initiative facing Western society. The disorder is more common than cancer and AIDS combined, and it is the mechanism by which we, in Western society, have created a new constellation of killer diseases from which we all suffer to a variable degree but increasingly so.

Our current lifestyle and behavior is largely responsible for this problem. Our lifestyle is sedentary, watching television, sitting in front of computers, and driving everywhere. Over the past century technological developments have almost completely removed physical exercise from our day-to-day lives. In association with diet, and mainly as a result of diet, this lifestyle sets the scene for the major killers outlined above. The problem now affects not only the elderly or even the middle-aged, it is also having major effects on children and teenagers.

Mankind has evolved over about four million years, but only in the last century has change developed at such an unrelenting pace never before experienced. We have walked the roads to and from our destinations day in, day out, for all these millions of years. In the past few thousand years, the fastest mode of transportation has been the horse. In the past century, we have developed the technology to travel the world in a day, from New York to Australia, and to drive vehicles at over 100 mph. We have become dependent upon mechanization in every walk of life, buses to school and cars to work; engines to dig and toil the soil, to build roads and buildings, and to manufacture goods. The effects of living in front of television and computer screens, and eating and drinking carbohydrate-laced foods, has been to create a new model of human. Our supermarket shelves are packed with cheap, mass-produced, good-tasting, readily available food, which is high in calories. These foods are attractively displayed in advertisements on televisions to which we have become glued.

People who migrate to the United States from poor areas such as Latin America and Asia adopt Western lifestyles and become obese. Improved nutrition has done much to enhance human performance, physical and possibly intellection performance, but modern nutrition has created the major killing diseases.

Eating our way through this mountain of sugar is the primary cause of heart attacks. Vascular disease, strokes, and diabetes, as well as breast cancer, uterine, and ovarian cancer are also associated with overeating. Inflammation of the liver, increased tendency for the blood to clot, and depression of the immune system are part of the equation as well. These disorders are created by twentieth and twenty-first century living. Admittedly, in the nineteenth century people died at a younger age, most often of infectious diseases such as tuberculosis or pneumonia, which have now been dramatically reduced by the innovations of antibiotics and vaccination. Vaccination has been the biggest life saver of all time.

In addition to the major killers, most gastrointestinal diseases, which are extremely common, are caused by the modern diet. These are gallstones, diverticular disease, appendicitis, hemorrhoids, and inflammatory bowel disease.

Our earliest ancestors ate foods similar to those eaten by apes and monkeys. These were fruits, shoots, nuts, tumors, and other vegetations in the forests of Africa. Most of these plants were relatively low in calories and took constant work to collect them and thus to stay alive. Early mankind began eating meat some two and a half million years ago, and the fossil record shows that the human brain became remarkably bigger and more complex at about this time. The incorporation of animal matter into the diet played an essential role in human evolution. The fatty acids found in meat also played an important role in brain growth.

Energy exists in many different forms; oil and food are forms of chemical energy. Burning oil permits planes to fly, cars to run, houses to be heated and cooled, and electricity to be generated. Burning food permits us to live, run, walk, talk, and do our many lifetime activities. The energy that isn't actively burned in a plane or a car is stored in the fuel tank. When the tanks are empty the vehicle stops. Oil is a form of fat, and in man, unused energy is stored as fat. When the fat stores are totally depleted, the subject dies as some fats are essential for life to continue.

Mankind derives energy from three sources: protein, carbohydrates, and fat. We are extremely efficient in the collection, storage, and utilization of energy, much more so than planes or cars. The energy taken in food is either utilized or not burned, the excess to be stored as fat. In the process of staying alive, maintaining our bodies, and our body temperatures, we use energy in the order of about 1500 calories per day. When we work, play sports and run, or partake in other activities, we burn up additional energy. We can utilize a maximum of about 3000 calories per day, but a huge Thanksgiving dinner can provide 6,000 calories, many more calories than can be expended even by running a marathon. Differences in calorific needs exist for men and women. Physical exercise, like riding a bicycle for an hour, typically burns only 300 to 400 calories, but exercise is important in the energy equation.

The body does not act as a storage organ for protein. Weightlifters and muscle men store some energy in their increased muscle mass but not a lot. Likewise, the body is a poor storage organ for carbohydrate.

There is some carbohydrate in muscle and about 150 grams in the liver, stored as the chemical glycogen. The body stores of glycogen are about 600 calories or the equivalent of about two hours of riding on the bike. Clearly, after two hours on the bike we do not show signs of massive energy depletion, so we start to utilize fat stores. These fat stores have the potential to be huge.

A morbidly obese person has basically the same frame size as a skinny person. They have the same amount of bone, a little more muscle, the same size brain, the same lungs and guts, and a little bigger heart. If the basic frame of a 600-pound man is 150 pounds, then he is carrying 450 pounds of fat and carrying it twenty-four hours a day—every time he moves, every time he walks, every time he climbs stairs. That is the equivalent of carrying four large sacks of grain on his back every time he moves. These sacks of grain strain the heart, the lungs, the muscles, the bones, and the joints and lead to the rapid development of cardiac and vascular disease.

If we eat an excess of 1000 calories per day, this will produce a weight gain of approximately 100 grams per day or about two pounds a week, which is 100 pounds a year. The balance of intake and utilization of energy is an accurate one, as according to the laws of thermodynamics energy cannot be created or destroyed elsewhere. Conversely, if someone is 100 pounds overweight, each pound of fat contains 3500 calories, so to reduce this you would need to save 350,000 calories, which on a 1000-calorie diet would take between one and two years.

The American Heart Association has for many years stated that eating saturated fats such as butter and lard will increase the process of arteriosclerosis. On the other hand, eating polyunsaturated fats is thought to help keep the arteries clear. Healthy intake of fats depends upon getting the correct proportion of the various fats in the diet. The modern Western diet has a serious imbalance in the ratio of omega-3 to omega-6 fatty acids. This is a result of consuming a lot of refined carbohydrates and relatively small amounts of omega-3 fatty acids. In contrast, for centuries, the source of essential fatty acids was omega-3-rich whole grains, nuts, vegetables, and even eggs.

Natives of Greenland traditionally live on a diet that consists of meat and blubber from seals and whales. These natives feed on fish whose flesh has a high concentration of omega-3 fatty acids. Omega-3 fatty acids lower triglycerides and LDL cholesterol. Furthermore, they lower blood pressure and have an anticoagulant effect, thus preventing coronary artery thrombosis and stroke. Heart disease is extremely rare in the classical indigenous Greenland native. Several studies have shown that eating fish reduces death from coronary artery disease. Between 2 and 3 percent of Greenlanders may carry a gene that protects them from gaining weight no matter how much sugar they eat. Scientists from the University of Copenhagen have discovered that these people ingest carbohydrates that are not absorbed into the blood. This results in them having a lower body mass index, fat percentage, and cholesterol levels. It is hoped that these findings will lead to a drug that balances sugar absorption and prevents obesity and heart disease.

It has been known since the 1950s that men over the age of thirty have a progressive increase in mortality with increasing weight. The increase begins with weights just in excess of the acceptable weight range but accelerates exponentially thereafter. Excess weight gain in females is also associated with increased mortality, but this begins at a somewhat older age than in men. It has been shown that if the obese lose weight they may again enter into an optimal range for longevity. This adds further evidence to the conclusion that obesity decreases lifespan. The other measurable factor that has a major influence on longevity is smoking. In nonsmoking men and women, the risk of being 35 to 50 percent overweight respectively confers the same risk as smoking with the body weight within the acceptable range. People are now smoking less, so there are more deaths attributed to excess weight than to smoking.

Obesity has been shown to have a significant role to play in the genesis of coronary artery disease. There are, however, other risk factors including age, male sex, hypertension, smoking, and elevated cholesterol concentrations.

Some of these other risk factors, particularly high blood pressure and serum cholesterol, are directly related to obesity. Another factor related to heart disease and obesity is physical inactivity, which has been scientifically shown in many studies to be related to the development of heart disease. It ultimately plays a role in obesity at all ages.

It has been shown that both vigorous exercise and walking are protective not only from the point of view of containing developing obesity, but also in preventing coronary artery disease. The exact mechanism of its protective effect is not fully understood, but the burning of calories goes some way towards achieving it. Obesity also creates hypertension, particularly with increasing age. Evidence also exists that a reduction in weight will reduce blood pressure. The relationship between obesity and diabetes is beyond question, and diabetes is a factor in the development of heart disease and hypertension.

Historically, and again considering the evolutionary pathway, consumption of meat, which produced a growth in the brain-produced guile, cunning, and organization, led to the development of community living, but the supply of this food required a lot of energy to be expended in catching the prey. This supply was sporadic and led to an overall lean body habitus, particularly as a result of food deprivation during the winters.

The American Cancer Society has shown an association between obesity and increased risk of cancer of the colon, rectum, and prostate. With increasing weight, women show a progressive increase in the risk of cancer of the breast, ovaries, uterus, and cervix.

Obesity places a considerable burden on the heart and respiratory system. Lung function becomes increasingly impaired with increasing weight, vis-à-vis carrying the sacks of grain referred to earlier. It further impairs exercise tolerance and, ultimately, the morbidly obese patient with the combination of heart, lung, and joint disease becomes beleaguered and totally unable to perform any form of exercise. Even walking or climbing stairs becomes severely restricted. Some become entrapped in their houses even being unable to get through the door!

Another very common problem in association with obesity is sleep apnea. Sleep apnea is a condition in which levels of oxygen within the bloodstream fall, leading to sleep fragmentation, frequent awakening, and eventually to the development of right-sided heart failure. This is associated with maladies of brain function and cognition, which may occur as a result of damage to the central nervous system. The course of this condition is chronic and progressive. Weight loss will, however, reverse the heart condition, but not the damage to the central nervous system.

Chapter 8
Obesity and Covid-19

Obesity is the major cause of death from Covid-19 infection. The development of the Covid-19 virus has been the greatest public health threat for over a century. It is undergoing various mutations, the most recent of which seem to increase its ability to infect the population at large. The virus has now killed well over a million people and the number affected has run into the billions; the figures are increasing in most countries of the world on a daily basis. We are currently, at the time of writing, experiencing an exponential growth in the prevalence of the Omicron variant of the virus. Previous pandemics have radically changed society and the economic consequences of Covid-19 have been huge. Fourteen million people in the United States lost their jobs, at least temporarily, and the stock markets have been in the state of flux, but have, in fact, been very resilient.

We are now entering a new and unforeseen outbreak of the latest variant, which perhaps produces a somewhat milder disease, and there could be more transitions. It has been forecast by the leading epidemiologist from Oxford University, Sarah Gilbert, that new pandemics unrelated to those of a coronavirus origin could arise in the future.

There has been a massive effect on world economies with the closure of many small businesses, particularly in the entertainment and retail business. Perhaps ironically there has been a rapid expansion in the availability of jobs, and there are more jobs available than those who are either adequately skilled or interested enough to take them up. The virus has undergone several mutations but the latest of these, the Omicron triple mutation, has raised the greatest scare as it is highly transmissible and is doubling after every two to three days. The actual overall relevance of this mutant remains to be determined, and it appears that it is less aggressive, in terms of hospitalization and producing deaths, than its preceding Delta variant. It does, however, appear to be overcoming the Delta variant as the major Covid-19 mutant producing disease across the world from South Africa, where it began, through to Western Europe and the United States.

This highly contagious virus affects all cross-sections of the community from children to the elderly. With the early forms of the disease, most children and adults up to middle age have experienced milder disease. The Omicron variant seems to have more of an affinity for infecting younger people and studies on its effect in the elderly, who are now highly protected, frequently from a triple vaccine, have not as yet been fully studied. We don't know the exact prevalence of the disease, as many cases are entirely asymptomatic but still transmissible. Nations produce annual figures and figures on a daily basis, but these figures are undoubtedly an underestimate as there is no way in accessing so many, probably millions of people, who are asymptomatic or develop the disease and lie in bed at home without communicating their illness to the various government authorities. The earliest forms of Covid-19 focused particularly on the elderly, many of whom have comorbidities exacerbated by the presence of the virus that led to their early death.

The major comorbidity that predisposes individuals to die from the virus is undoubtedly obesity. Other comorbidities also related to obesity are diabetes, heart disease, and hypertension, all of which can be caused by excess weight. Covid-19 has been the major, worldwide killer this year, but it has also had a profound effect on deaths from the other major killers, as access to hospitalization and adequate methods of intensive care treatment have been blocked by the saturation of beds with those who suffer from Covid-19 and frequently require long-term ventilation and often after months on a ventilator subsequently succumb to the disease.

The Covid-19 lockdown fueled an alarming rise in childhood obesity. Twenty-five percent of children aged ten to eleven years are now obese, compared with 20 percent before the pandemic, but equally concerning is that 41 percent are classified as being overweight.

Obesity in four and five-year-olds has risen by 50 percent in the last twenty years, and of those beginning school, 14.4 percent were obese in 2021 compared with 10 percent in 2019. These figures are based on the UK National Child Measurement Program that weighs 300,000 school pupils. It has recorded by far the biggest rise in childhood obesity since the program was started, placing obesity in children at an all-time high, and raising the incidence of type II diabetes in children to an unprecedented level and even increasing childhood cancer, thus increasing the risk of early death from all of the major killers.

Constraints are now being placed on junk food advertising and clinics are being set up to advise parents and children. During the lockdown it appears that children confined to home have been endlessly snacking on junk food in addition to eating their normal meals, and they have been prevented from getting out with friends and burning calories using exercise. In addition, the quality of school meals has declined and healthy meal provision has gone out of the window. It is essential that measures are taken to break the junk food cycle, its advertising, and its prominent display at supermarket checkouts. Boys have developed a higher prevalence of obesity than girls across all ages, and children living in socially deprived areas are twice as commonly affected as those in more middle-class environments. Once a child is obese, it is highly likely that this child will stay obese for life.

A summary of the evidence so far suggests that obesity is associated with the highest risk of developing the severe symptoms and complications independent of all other illnesses such as cardiovascular disease.

The Centers for Disease Control and Prevention (CDC) strongly emphasizes that severe obesity is the single most important factor in the progression of Covid-19 disease from what might be a relatively mild disorder to a disease resulting in hospitalization, long periods of ventilator dependence, and ultimately death, predominantly from pneumonia.

Those people with obesity frequently have other medical problems, in particular hypertension. Recent studies, however, point to obesity in itself as the most significant factor in necessitating hospitalization that occurs due to the Covid-19 virus. This may be because obesity is a proinflammatory disease that may exacerbate the production of cytokines, themselves a major contributing factor to multiple organ failure, the major killer in Covid-19 disease. The World Health Organization and the World Obesity Federation have emphasized this danger. Those countries with extremely high rates of obesity like the USA have suffered badly from the disease and the numbers are still rising. The same is true to a slightly lesser extent in Britain, and once the obese patient with Covid-19 becomes ventilator dependent they may remain on the ventilator for weeks and ultimately develop pneumonia leading to multiple organ failure and death. The mortality under these circumstances in the ventilator-dependent obese patient is between 80 and 88 percent. This startling example emphasizes the importance of overcoming obesity.

At the time of writing, Covid-19 is not yet over and may continue to produce more deaths for many years and be with us perhaps permanently. The lifestyle impaired by Covid-19 can be debilitating and unhealthy, producing lack of exercise, overeating, depression, and isolation. Manifestations of the disease in patients with long Covid, which may be expected to last for many years, may require multiple frequent vaccinations being necessary to keep it under control, though as yet we do not know the ultimate outcome. It is of interest, however, that the Spanish flu of 1918 underwent multiple mutations and ultimately burned itself out by becoming more mild with subsequent mutations. Perhaps we can only hope that this will be the case with Covid-19; the reason for this is that the virus needs to continue to infect people to survive and if the more aggressive forms of the disease are blocked by the vaccine, further mutations will be required and these mutations may, hopefully, in the long run, lead to the development of a less clinically severe disease. This may be the case as the disease appears to be diminishing in South Africa where it first was recognized.

The future is one of high financial costs for years to come. Undoubtedly, the pandemic will continue. The new variant Omicron will perhaps further mutate and produce additional changes that may make the vaccines less effective, and there are groups of research virologists now working on a new, modified vaccine to control the Omicron outbreak.

The evidence available in mid 2022 suggests that the Omicron infection is generally milder than the Delta variant and may damage the lungs less than Delta and the previous original Wuhan strain. According to research by Cambridge University, Omicron appears less efficient at infecting cells in the deep parts of the lungs, which had a vulnerability to the other varieties of the disease that led to severe life-threatening illness.

Encouragingly, existing reports from South Africa have shown that there is surprisingly little serious disease with the Omicron variant and fewer hospitalizations and deaths. The United States and UK are presently experiencing daily increases in the number of cases, which seem to be frequently doubling. It is possible that the indigenous immunity between the South African population and that in Western countries is different, though this is currently unknown. It appears that the risk factors for the newer serious variant of the disease are the same, principally obesity and type II diabetes. The benefit of vaccination is that it speeds up the body's immune response and makes it more likely that the immune system will win the race before the serious forms of the disease develop.

Early data suggests that symptoms of Omicron are more similar to those of a common cold with a runny nose, headache, and fatigue together with sneezing and sore throat, rather than the classic Covid symptoms, such as loss of taste and smell and severe weakness. This may be because Omicron varies much more widely from the preexisting variants having fifty mutations including thirty-two in the SDG, the gene that encodes the virus's spike protein that allows it to access our cells. This varies much more than the Delta gene, which does contain the S gene. It is possible that the presence of colds and flu and other winter viruses, by raising their own antibodies, may be protective against the Omicron, limiting the amount of the virus that can accumulate in the tissues.

The symptoms following infection with Omicron appear much quicker, usually about two days after contact, but they seem to last less time, typically two and a half to three days. It is, however, possible that the Omicron variant is able to avoid some of the immunity found efficacious against the Alpha and Delta variants. The good news is that the symptoms on the whole do appear to be less severe. The big plus appears to be that the booster jab increases protection to more than 70 percent after previously having two shots of the vaccine. This is because the boosters stimulate the body into making more antibodies than the quantity of antibodies you have gained in the system, which could count in regard to resistance to any new coming variant. A further fact is that killer T cells are triggered by the vaccine, and they can target the virus when it is a new variant and are not entirely focused on the spike protein. Unfortunately, the disease still occurs in people who have been triple vaccinated.

This will not be the last time we will face a life-threatening virus. There will be more. We must diversify vaccine development and manufacture these vaccines as quickly as possible. To combat a new pandemic, the Service Center in Oxford is combining a multi-professional strategy with virologists and immunologists working with industry. This rapidly increases the progress that can be made to fight multiple viruses. Currently, drugs have been developed that are effective in the treatment of the disease. There are other new areas where vaccine development has made a huge breakthrough, particularly in the field of malaria.

CHAPTER 9
OBESITY AND LIFE EXPECTANCY

The future forecasts a potential decline in life expectancy as a result of obesity.

Projections of life expectancy form an important component of government strategy with regard to such programs as Social Security and Medicare. Until recently, all forecasts of life expectancy favored a continuing increase in longevity. As stated, for the past thousand years there has been a slow and steady increase in life expectancy, occasionally changed by epidemics, famines, and major wars. The risk of major pandemics still exists. This declined after the influenza outbreak at the end of World War I that killed over two million people, more than were killed in the war, but clearly major risks still exist, as with the development of the latest and possibly one of the greatest pandemics, the Covid-19 pandemic. Irrespective of pandemics, gains in life expectancy have been stunted, and in some cases, there has been a decline from where they were in the first decade of the twenty-first century. The main cause of this is eating disorders.

Some prognostications of life expectancy have been overoptimistic. The United Nations forecasted a projected life expectancy of 100 years for males and females in developed countries by the year 2300. Furthermore, the Social Security Administration arrived at a figure of life expectancy reaching the mid-eighties by the middle of this century.

These forecasts are now being seriously questioned as a result of the unprecedented increase in obesity in Western countries and the development of pandemics, of which there may be more in the future.

If current trends continue, they will undoubtedly threaten to diminish the health and life expectancy of current and future generations. As has been stated, two thirds of adults in the United States today are obese or overweight and 50 percent of African Americans are currently obese. An article in The New England Journal of Medicine reports that children and ethnic minorities have shown the greatest increase in obesity, and this is likely to persist with them throughout life. These trends have affected all major racial and ethnic groups and all socioeconomic strata and have been particularly marked in those of lower socioeconomic status.

It has now been estimated that obesity causes approximately a quarter of a million deaths per year in the United States. The risk of developing diabetes in the United States has risen exponentially to a figure of about 40 percent. The life-shortening effect of diabetes is approximately thirteen years. If the prevalence of obesity continues to rise, it will lead to an elevated risk of associated morbidities with a negative outcome. The reason so many people become obese now is that, in the long term, they ingest more calories than their needs. This surfeit of calories, whether taken in the form of carbohydrate or fat, results in the accumulation within the body of excess fat cells. People who are obese not only have more fat cells present in their bodies, which amount to several trillion, but the fat cells themselves become enlarged.

Obesity often begins early in life and reduces life expectation by increasing the incidence and aggression of all of the other major killers outlined in this text. A continued rise in the prevalence of obesity could, for the first time in the thousand years, lead to a statistical downturn in longevity for the whole population.

It is impossible to predict the ultimate outcome of the Covid19 pandemic or indeed to forecast the likelihood of other and potentially more fatal pandemics in the future. There are other realistic existing threats to increases in life expectancy, such as an increase in the AIDS epidemic and the resurgence of mutations of the influenza virus like SARS, MERS, and H1N1, all of which have killed tens of thousands in the last twenty years. Infectious diseases have always, over the past century, presented the greatest threat to life expectation and they may still do so. Another major threat in the past has been famine, but now for the first time, the major and probable inevitable threat to increased longevity relates directly to the presence of obesity and an excess of available food rather than starvation. Suffice it to say that we cannot forecast the devastating effect that a nuclear war might have, and this cannot be discounted in view of the increasing threats placed on Western countries by China and Russia.

CHAPTER 10
REASONS FOR OBESITY

Why do people become obese?

People become obese because, in the long term, they ingest more calories, significantly in excess of their needs. Whether these are in the form of excess carbohydrate, which is the most common, or fat, they gain fat cells within their body to an amazing extent that is largely unlimited.

Obesity often begins early in life. There has been a doubling in the incidence of obesity in three and four-year-old children in the last decade and this has further accelerated with the quarantine periods and school closures of the Covid-19 era. During this time there has been no change in birth weight and of course no change in the gene pool; thus, obesity in children is acquired and relates primarily to present-day lifestyle. Factors that contribute to this are the following: the increased consumption of fatty foods and high calorie carbohydrate drinks, reduced physical activity brought on by television viewing and computer games, food advertising, abandonment of breastfeeding. These factors are strongly influenced by parents who it must be said are largely to blame.

A major factor in this vicious equation is advertising, which is extremely powerful. Food marketeers target children and adults to influence their food choices on their eating behavior. So lucrative is this business that large companies contract to provide free computers and televisions to schools in exchange for compelling the children to view two minutes of commercial messages each day. Food advertising makes up a large proportion of this viewing time. This perhaps reflects on the way in which the nation's schools are funded. In relative terms, education has become increasingly poorly financed. Furthermore, the effectiveness of advertising campaigns are surreptitious and difficult to evaluate. We are all immersed in a sea of advertising, to a much greater degree than we are aware. If advertising was not so influential, companies would not invest in it, but observation of the plethora of advertising on television, the Internet, and their prevalence on our screens, only goes to emphasize what is the focal point and what a huge relevance it has in our everyday life, and we are all, whether we would admit to it or not, highly subject to it and influenced by it.

In the past decade, in some school districts, fast food companies took over school food service operations. Under these circumstances, the fast food company eliminates the burden to the school of providing meals that the child will eat. The question of appropriate nutrition, physical activity, and weight management never enters the equation. These meal services are often supplemented by vending machines that provide an endless supply of sugar-soaked sodas, which are accessible throughout the day.

Over the past decade soda sales to school distributors increased by over 1000 percent. Each can of soda contains the equivalent of ten teaspoons of sugar. One large soda drink can supply one half of the total daily calorie counts required by a teenager. The average child consumes in excess of one can of soda per day. A correlation exists between soda consumption and obesity in childhood. Soda consumption combined with an increasing lack of exercise is a potent combination in the production of obesity.

The above social factors driving obesity in childhood have been generated by, and are equally present in, the adult. Adults and children walk less, ride in more cars, and use more public transport than ever before. There are more elevators, escalators, conveyor belts, televisions, computers, iPhones, and the equivalent and more couches. Conversely, there are more gymnasiums, sales of exercise equipment, jogging tracks, and other sports facilities. These latter, however, are only used by a small cross-section of the community, but because of the physical encumbrance produced by their excess fat, obese and morbidly obese patients are unable to use these aids or take advantage of them.

The exact mechanism by which man controls his energy intake in order to maintain a steady weight is not fully understood. A "set point" seems to exist that, in practical terms, is a buffer zone around which most people manage to keep their weight fairly stable over the years. It is possible for the body to reset the set point in an upward direction so that the prolonged and continuous access to the intake of food will produce elevation of this point of equilibrium. On the other hand, defense of the set point has been used to explain why the maintenance of medically induced weight loss has turned out to be so poor and why weight loss programs have almost inevitably failed.

Energy conservation is a factor that influences short-term weight stability. So often one hears from patients that they have virtually starved for several days but not lost any weight. When fasting the body enters a conservation mode, this results in a reduction of energy output by reducing metabolic rate to compensate for the sudden shutdown of food intake, rather like the mechanism that underlies hibernation in mammals. This mechanism is probably not only confined to energy intake but also to energy usage by the body, for exercise in day-to-day activities. Such conservation is probably related to the short-term stabilizing factor produced by the set point, and longer periods of starvation are needed to start the weight reduction sequence.

The storage of fat in mammals and later in man has evolved over millions of years as a primary mechanism for coping with, initially, food deprivation in winter, and perhaps later, periods of famine. For most of the four million years that man has existed on this planet, the major problem was getting enough food to eat. In the average adult, there is something around fifty to one hundred billion fat cells. Losing weight causes the fat cells to shrink in size and to become less metabolically active, but their number only goes down very slowly, which is perhaps why people who have lost large amounts of weight end up with their skin sagging and underlying depleted fat cells giving them something of a fatty apron over their abdomen. Hibernation in animals involves the process of fat storage and slow usage, which maintains life throughout the winter.

The process of inflammation is currently receiving increasing attention. Fat cells promote inflammation, which can spread throughout the body. Even small amounts of excess fat can produce a mounting immune response. This is because the body regards the storage of excess fat cells as an invading foreign organism and attempts to reject its presence by mounting up an inflammatory response. Inflammation is now viewed as a key mechanism in the development of heart disease, probably being more important than the accumulation of cholesterol per se. Blood vessels such as the coronary arteries are undoubtedly narrowed by cholesterol, as previously stated, but the big problem appears to be that of an inflamed plaque that can break open and upon which blood clot can settle and occlude the vessel, producing thrombosis and the cutoff of oxygen to the tissue involved. In the case of the coronary arteries, this leads to the death of heart muscle and commonly to death. Compounds secreted by fat cells contribute to vascular inflammation and inhibit nitric oxide, a compound that helps relax blood vessel walls and lowers blood pressure, conversely leading to hypertension. Fat cells also secrete estrogen, which is linked to certain types of cancer such as prostate, breast, ovarian, and uterine cancer. Researchers now suspect that the origin of diabetes also lies at least in part in the biochemistry of fat in the production of inflammation. These substances involved in this mechanism are referred to as resistin and tumor necrosis factor-alpha. Inflammation is an important aspect relating to health and longevity and is considered further below.

Fat cells behave differently in different parts of the body. Fat carried in the hips and thighs is considered to be comparatively benign, whereas that which accumulates around the organs of the abdomen is more harmful, and this is more common in males than females. This fat around the abdomen is metabolically more active and produces more inflammation, thus promoting clots, than is the case with fat distributed around the periphery of the body. Fortunately, visceral fat is the first to disappear in response to exercise, a key point in favor of taking regular exercise. The actual distribution of body fat is genetically determined, but the amount of fat stored relates directly to excess intake over output.

CHAPTER 11
THE EFFECT THAT TECHNOLOGY HAS HAD ON LIFESTYLE

As has been stated, the congregation of early mankind into cities, towns, and villages coincided with the invention of controlled agriculture. This provided a steady and predictable source of food, which could be replenished through the seasons and stored in the winter. The shift from wild meat and vegetation to cultivated grains, however, deprived humans of many of the essential amino acids, vitamins, and minerals upon which they had thrived for the preceding millions of years. Although these advances increased lifespan and perhaps brainpower, average height diminished, and dental caries and bone disorders became apparent for the first time. These were due to nutritional deficiencies that had started to manifest themselves in skeletal remains and with them bacterial infections increased. At this time, however, obesity was not a problem, and this remained the situation until about 100 years ago when the technological revolution led to a reduced need for hard physical labor. Improved technology has made crops of grain and dairy products both cheaper to produce and more plentiful. But along with these changes has come the bubble of obesity, which is now culminating in a reduction in life expectation for the first time in centuries.

In the United States wealthy people tend to be thinner than those of lower socioeconomic status. One in three living below the poverty line is obese compared with one in six in the households with an income in excess of $70,000 per year. In addition, obesity is more common in African Americans and minority ethnic groupings. This is probably down to eating the wrong foods, and children in particular are prone to do this. The availability of junk food has increased exponentially and, in its promulgation, the power of advertising cannot be underestimated. It has now been estimated that in the United States approximately 50 percent of food budgets are spent in restaurants or on takeouts. Here, in order to make the supersize meals more tasty and attractive, additional fats and carbohydrates are added. They also add to food preservation. Unfortunately, this type of food is stacked with the unhealthy trans fatty acids.

Chapter 12
Psychological Factors

We are living through extremely stressful times, not only with the pandemic, but with economic instabilities, inflation, unemployment, and living through periods of isolation and quarantine. Psychiatric problems are commonly associated with poor eating and subsequently in the development of the obese state. It is hardly surprising that the morbidly obese individual, who cannot climb a flight of stairs, sit in the normal seat, wear conventional clothes, or get on a bus or a plane would have low self-esteem. Low self-esteem leads to social isolation. Many of these people refuse to go out of the house in the daytime and they make essential visits to the supermarket after dark. This sort of social isolation produces depression, and food provides solace for the depressed. They then return home and eat the cheapest, most unhealthy foods purchased from the supermarket and gain more weight. This forms the basis of all of the major killers discussed in this book.

Societies across the nations have developed an antagonistic attitude toward obesity. Obese children tend to be disliked, looked down upon, and regarded as figures of fun. Their obese state is associated with shame, and they are thought to be self-indulgent and lacking in willpower. They are also thought to be responsible for their condition, whereas children with other physical disabilities are not, and they usually receive sympathy and support. A majority of these obese children have obese parents and social and family pressures can lead to overeating as it is often regarded as a sign of appreciation to eat as much as possible of the food presented and not to waste any. All parties and celebrations are based on the provision of food and such practices are societal. Most major social events are based around eating, at least a small feast, and such practices have gone on since before Roman times, and the eating of food has thus become an important ritual, and its excess can lead to addiction.

The more obese the subject becomes the greater is the incidence of depression. A number of factors contribute to the development of psychological problems that culminate in chronic depression: there is low self-worth, reduced quality of life, inefficiency at work, impaired sexual relationships, and social isolation. Perhaps, on the other hand, a woman who was sexually abused in childhood may purposely attempt to gain weight to make herself less attractive to men. Employment may be difficult to obtain for those who are obese. Over two thirds of obese patients report abuse: physical, 34 percent; sexual, 12 percent; and psychological, 64 percent. One third of morbidly obese patients report a family history of alcoholism. On the other hand, alcoholism in the morbidly obese subject is relatively rare.

It has been known since the 1950s that men between the ages of thirty and thirty-nine have a progressive increase in mortality with increasing weight. The increase begins with weights just in excess of the acceptable weight range. The overall mortality in obese men increases with age thereafter.

Excess weight gain in the female is also associated with increased mortality, which begins at a somewhat older age than in men. Those overweight men and women who lose substantial amounts of weight and remain at a weight within the optimal range for an appreciable amount of time appear to have a lower mortality risk than an equivalent group of overweight individuals. This adds further evidence to the conclusion that obesity decreases lifespan. Obesity has been shown to have a significant role to play in the genesis of coronary artery disease. There are, however, other strong risk factors including age, male sex, hypertension, smoking, and elevated cholesterol concentrations.

Most of these risk factors, particularly hypertension and high serum cholesterol, are a direct result of obesity. Another factor related to heart disease and obesity is physical inactivity, which has been scientifically shown in many studies to be related to the development of heart disease.

It ultimately plays a role in obesity at all ages. It has been shown that both vigorous exercise and walking are protective not only from the point of view of containing developing obesity, but also coronary artery disease. The exact mechanism of the protective effect is not fully understood, but it does seem to relate to calorific intake. Studies on the whole of obesity are somewhat conflicting, but there is good evidence as weight increases with increasing age, there is an elevation of blood pressure. In addition, evidence exists that weight loss results in a reduction in blood pressure. The relationship between obesity and diabetes is beyond question, and diabetes is also a factor in the development of heart disease and hypertension.

Chapter 13
Alzheimer's Disease

Alzheimer's disease is the most common cause of dementia in the Western world. Dementia is a name of a group of symptoms associated with an ongoing decline of brain function. It can affect primarily memory, but also thinking skills, and can interfere with day-to-day abilities and maintaining an independent life. The exact cause of Alzheimer's disease is not fully understood, although there are pointers towards an explanation of the problem. The first is Alzheimer's disease is a disease of increasing age and is more common in those with depression and those with a family history of Alzheimer's disease. It has been projected to triple in incidence over the next twenty-five years and to become the major killer in Western countries.

Alzheimer's disease is the major cause of dementia, which may also be due to other factors and is associated with diet, cardiovascular disease, cholesterol levels, high blood sugar concentrations and diabetes, hypertension, lack of exercise, and smoking. Smoking, currently a major factor, is marked by a declining incidence in society so the major identifiable factor probably responsible for a tripling of the incidence of the disease in the future is, again, related to diet you eat.

Head injury in sport is now regarded as another major cause of dementia. This has caused great concern among players and administrators in the NFL and the European football leagues where brain damage is due to either head-to-head contact in American football or repeated heading of the ball in the Premier League and the European football leagues. Worldwide about fifty million people suffer from dementia. The estimated proportion of the general population aged sixty and over with dementia is about 8 percent, a figure which rises with increasing age. It is not an inevitable consequence of aging. Many people over the age of 100 are alert, clear thinking, and have an excellent recall.

Alzheimer's disease is associated with a buildup of deposits of a protein named amyloid, which is distributed throughout the brain. These plaques surround brain cells slowly destroying them. A second protein called "tau" also becomes tangled within brain cells. Alzheimer's disease may begin relatively early in life before any symptoms become apparent and it goes on for many years, slowly affecting the brain cells and interfering with neurotransmission that sends messages or signals between brain cells. There appears to be a low level of one neurotransmitter, acetylcholine, in the brains of patients with Alzheimer's disease. The disease leads to a shrinkage of the brain with loss of cells. The areas of the brain affected vary from case to case and several different forms of Alzheimer's disease exist, some of which, for example, predominantly affect the visual cortex and lead to impairment of vision and possibly blindness. The most common early symptom, however, is loss of short-term memory. Most patients retain their long-term memory in great detail and can recount early episodes of their lives with absolute accuracy, but they frequently forget either the names of colleagues and friends or even what they had to eat for breakfast. Loss of memory, for example for names, is an accepted manifestation of aging in the elderly—we all get it!

Age is a single most significant factor in the disease, and it increasingly occurs, doubling every five years, beyond the age of sixty-five. It is, however, not only the very elderly who suffer from Alzheimer's disease and it often occurs at an earlier stage in life.

Brain damage occurs in association with different careers. An issue that has become increasingly concerning is the number of people who develop dementia at an early age following head injuries after playing either in the NFL, rugby or soccer. In the NFL it has been put down to head injuries, sustained from head-to-head contact during the game as a result of head butting, and in soccer it has been attributed to the daily repeated multiple episodes of heading the ball. Head injuries, either in the NFL or in football associated with heading the ball, occur as a result of the brain being pushed backwards and forwards within the bony cranium and sustaining damage as it impacts against the inner bony lining of the skull.

Genetic factors also seem to a play a part in developing Alzheimer's disease and in a few families, it seems to be related to the inheritance of a single gene and the risk of the condition being passed on by this.

Research has shown that several lifestyle factors are associated with the onset of Alzheimer's disease: diet, cardiovascular disease, obesity, diabetes, hypertension, high cholesterol, and smoking. Once again, these factors are those underlying the major causes of premature death today; they all have the same origins and they all can be ameliorated by an adjustment in diet. The purpose of this book is to highlight these factors and to emphasize their commonality because people can exercise, and cardiac and respiratory fitness lower the risk and slow the progression of the disease. In a large study in France people over the age of sixty-five were tested for the above parameters and then monitored for an average of eight and a half years. For every single item of the above seven factors, all of which are most significantly affected by dementia, for those who passed as healthy the risk of developing dementia went down by 10 percent for each. The study clearly demonstrates the link between diet, cardiovascular health, and the resilience of the brain with exactly the same triggering factors as those which occur with the other major killers. Thus, the risk of dementia can be reduced by a healthy lifestyle and eating the right types of food. Age remains a factor in the equation, but age per se is not the major or even an essential factor in developing dementia. What is good for the heart, therefore, is good for the brain. The risk factors are present for many years and begin in early life, so it is never too early to modify lifestyle accordingly and take the right steps to reduce the risk, primarily eating the right diet, taking steady exercise, staying mentally active, and being socially engaged.

As we age the brain normally starts to change by sixty, the frontal lobes and hippocampus, the areas involved in cognitive function and memory start to shrink, as does the white matter, the bundles of nerves that carry the signals between brain cells. With age the brain also carries fewer chemical messengers, including the feel-good hormones dopamine and serotonin, which can hasten depression and cognitive declines, ultimately contributing to Alzheimer's disease. Regular exercise is beneficial because it works at the cellular level to increase the number of mitochondria, the power units, in brain cells. Atmospheric pollution such as exhaust fumes and smoke from fires can lead to inflammation, cellular damage, and death if you run outside in the city center.

The major known precipitating factor relates again to the diet that we eat, and this is an essential factor in maintaining good brain function. It is more significant than genetics, which contributes 10 percent. Therefore, 90 percent appears to be down to lifestyle. The fundamental consideration in lifestyle is down to diet, which is the essential factor for adequate genetic function. Interestingly, the factors that contribute to the maintenance of brain function are essentially those that have been discussed in terms of cardiovascular disease, diabetes, and all of the other major killers. There are additional essential requirements for the more complex brain. The brain is particularly vulnerable to a poor diet. Brain cells continuously turn over and the breakdown of proteins and amino acids help to form new brain cells. In addition to protein, vegetables, fruit, and whole green grains supply energy to the brain cells. Omega-3, and to a lesser extent omega-6 fatty acids, contribute to the structure of cellular linings. Trans fats are again bad news as are refined sugars. It is the eating of more fast foods, rich in the latter, that is contributing the most to the rapid increase in Alzheimer's disease. Studies from Norway based on 30,000 people have shown that those who increased their lung function through exercise had a 40 to 50 percent reduced risk of developing Alzheimer's disease. The reason is that exercise causes complex chemical changes in the blood that affect the brain and slow down age-related diseases, including Alzheimer's. Recent studies are involving the transfusion of blood from young athletes after heavy exercise to those with Alzheimer's disease.

Today, well over 50 percent of new cases of dementia either have a vascular or a mixed vascular and Alzheimer's cause. Structured lifestyle intervention over time can dramatically diminish cognitive decline. At least 40 percent of dementia is preventable. Practical changes to diet, stress levels, sleep routine, and activity with social interaction can slow down its progress. Just twenty minutes of brisk walking per day can facilitate information processing and memory function.

Looking to the future, because vascular disease can play a major role in cognitive decline, it has recently been suggested that an ultrasound scan of the blood vessels in the neck can predict dementia ten years before the symptoms appear. Measuring the degree of arterial impairment through the carotid arteries in the neck can predict vascular damage to the brain, which impairs memory and thinking skills. Vascular disease in the neck due to hypertension can produce damage to very small, fragile vessels that supply the brain, often causing small bleeds, which can destroy brain cells causing memory and thinking problems and even minor strokes. Three thousand people were studied over a fifteen-year period with a measurement of their high intensity carotid pulse at the beginning of the study and an assessment of their cognitive capacity at the end. Those with carotid artery disease and a high intensity pulse were 50 percent more likely to have accelerated cognitive decline. This is an easily measurable and potentially treatable cause of cognitive decline in middle-aged individuals that can be spotted in advance and corrected. No major breakthroughs have otherwise been made in the treatment of established dementia. Researchers from Washington University medical school in 2019 described a blood test that is 94 percent accurate in detecting Alzheimer's disease many years before people develop memory loss and confusion. This advance could prove to be fundamentally important, not only in the detection, but ultimately in the treatment of this major killing disease of the elderly.

Drinking two cups of tea or two cups of coffee a day could reduce the risk of getting dementia by more than 25 percent. Scientists have found that while both of these drinks were individually linked to lowering the chances of either having a stroke or developing a memory disorder, consuming a combination of the two appeared to provide the greatest benefit. In the UK, 365,000 people were asked to record their coffee and tea intake and were followed for a period of fifteen years. Those who drank two cups of coffee and two cups of tea daily had a 28 percent lower risk of developing dementia than those who drank neither. They also had a 32 percent lower risk of sustaining a stroke. Drinking tea and coffee after a stroke halts the risks of dementia following the stroke. Plant chemicals such as flavonoids could explain the benefit incurred. A type of medicine that can help keep dementia at bay is medication for high blood pressure. People with untreated high blood pressure are more likely to have a stroke and develop cognitive decline. Loss of brain cells can be slowed by attempting to prevent inflammation, which is linked to depression and dementia. Plant flavonoids found in peppers, aubergines or eggplants, and green vegetables have anti-inflammatory, antiviral and antitumor activities.

Researchers using human, instead of simulated animal data, have discovered that Alzheimer's disease develops in a different way than was previously thought. These observations could have implications for new treatments.

Workers at Cambridge University have found that instead of developing from a single point in the brain, the disease develops in different unrelated areas simultaneously and separately. The speed with which it progresses depends on how quickly it destroys brain cells in these different regions. This occurs as a result of the production of toxic protein clusters.

These observations came from postmortem material as well as from PET scans from living patients with the disease. The damage to these different and unpredictable areas determines whether the disease develops rapidly or more slowly and how much cognitive impairment is produced. This relates to the aggregation of tau, one of the two key proteins implicated in the condition.

Tau and another toxic protein, amyloid-beta, buildup and entangle brain cells, and plaques form as aggregates causing their death producing shrinkage of the brain.

This results in memory loss, personality changes and a deterioration in the performance of day-to-day functions. The progression of the disease is dependent upon the replication of these aggregates in adjacent and different areas of the brain and not in the expansion of the disease from one area to another. The progress was previously thought to be a cascade, or a chain reaction, and this is no longer the case.

Early research was based on animal studies that produced different effects when toxic protein clusters were found in different parts of the brain. This was initially thought to be like a cancer, which spreads by local invasion. Instead, it is now shown to develop in multiple different areas of the brain so that trying to stop the spread from one region to another will do little to stop the progression of the disease. The focus of analysis needs to be at a molecular level of individual patients studied by PET scanning.

Deposits of tau aggregates is an extremely slow process taking up to five or more years; neurons are resistant to the damaging effects of tau and a focus needs to be made on slowing the process down further. The technology is evolving to stop the aggregation of proteins. This technology could also be applied to Parkinson's disease. The key discovery required is that stopping the replication of aggregates rather than the propagation is going to provide a more effective approach. This strategy could also be applied in the treatment of post-traumatic brain injury, as witnessed in football, NFL, and in rugby players.

The exact cause of Alzheimer's disease is not known; a number of factors, however, are considered to increase the risk. These are cardiovascular disease and obesity that place Alzheimer's in the same category of disease for which a major risk factor is a bad diet and obesity. Here again, regular exercise cardiac and respiratory fitness can lower the risk and slow the progression of the disease.

Chapter 14
Memory and the Effects of Diet

As people reach the age of sixty-five years, they naturally begin to forget things, like people's names and where they put things. These are the normal effects of aging and are not specifically signs of Alzheimer's disease

Harvard nutritionist and brain expert Dr. Uma Naidoo avoids five foods that weaken memory and focus. Despite advancing years it is never too late to act in a way that gives you the best possible chance of staving off dementia and making sure that you remain focused and smart. The Harvard scientist and author of This Is Your Brain on Food studied how gut bacteria can trigger metabolic processes and brain inflammation that can affect memory. Existing studies indicate that we may be able to reduce the possibility of dementia by avoiding foods that can compromise our gut bacteria and weaken our memory. Here are the foods that she tries to avoid in order to fight inflammation and promote brain health and function.

1. Added Sugars

The brain derives its energy from glucose, which fuels cellular activities. However, a high sugar diet can lead to excess glucose in the brain leading to memory impairment in functioning of the hippocampus, the memory controlling part of the brain.

2. Sodas

Sodas are loaded with refined sugars that rapidly hit the brain with too much glucose. The American Heart Association recommends that women consume no more than twenty-five grams of added sugars per day, and in men no more than thirty-six grams.

3. Fried Foods

Fried foods like French fries, tempura, samosas, fish and chips, and chicken fried steak should be avoided as much as possible. A study including 18,080 people found that a diet high in fried food was linked to lower scores in learning and memory. The most likely reason for this is that these foods cause inflammation that damages the small blood vessels in the brain. Another study of 715 people measured levels of depression and mental resilience and documented their levels of fried food consumption. Those who consume the most fried food were more likely to develop depression in their life. Ironically, avoiding fried foods can make you happier.

4. High Carbohydrate Foods

High carbohydrate foods, such as bread and pasta made from refined flour, are processed by the body in the same way as refined carbohydrates, and these are the carbohydrates that you need to avoid. It has been shown that these particular carbohydrates were associated with depression. In this study of 15,500 patients, better quality carbohydrates were defined as whole grains, foods higher in fiber, and those with a low glycemic index. These large molecule carbohydrates are the ones you need to add to your diet. The glycemic index is a measure of how quickly foods can convert to glucose when broken down during digestion. The faster the food is broken down to glucose the higher the glycemic index, and this is damaging. In this study those who ate better quality carbohydrates where 30 percent less likely to develop depression than those eating high glycemic carbohydrates. High glycemic index carbohydrates include potatoes, white bread, and white rice. Honey, orange juice, and whole meal breads are medium glycemic index foods. Low glycemic index foods are green vegetables, fruits, raw carrots, kidney beans, chickpeas and lentils. Blueberries contain antiaging properties, including better heart health and delayed cognitive aging. They are the best form of nutrition.

Chapter 15
Vaccination

Immunization is a global health and developmental success story, which saves millions of lives each year. Vaccines reduce the risk of getting a disease by working with the body's natural defenses to build protection. Vaccination increases the immune response to a disease by creating antibodies and proliferating T cells.

The multiple vaccines now available to the public currently prevent two to three million deaths every year, and that figure excludes the current impact of the vaccination for Covid.

Vaccines are essential in the control and elimination of over twenty potentially deadly diseases and in preventing further outbreaks. Access to vaccines worldwide is limited and many, in countries where they seem to be essential, do not have access. Additionally, a major problem that has arisen, particularly in the light of Covid-19 vaccination, is a resistance from the public, who with their children have an attitude to the vaccine and refuse it because of perceived potential side effects, which are often grossly exaggerated and are dishonestly presented on the Internet.

The major vaccines available today that have been shown to be effective in stimulating immunity to, and preventing infections from, these diseases are diphtheria, tetanus, pertussis, Covid-19, influenza, pneumococcus, Haemophilus influenza, measles, mumps, rubella, chickenpox, shingles, human papilloma virus, and hepatitis A, B, and C.

Immunization saves millions of lives each year by stimulating the immune response to the vaccine and preventing the development of the disease. This is a key component of primary health care, and it has saved more lives than any other branch of medicine and is the most effective healthcare investment available. The World Health Organization (WHO) has warned of an alarming decline in the number of children around the world receiving vaccines. This has precipitously declined particularly during the Covid-19 pandemic. Even when vaccines are available, there has been a marked increase in people refusing to receive them for themselves and their children. The problem of vaccine resistance is greatest in India, Pakistan, Southeast Asia, and Latin American countries where one could argue that they are most needed. The WHO provides global leadership in public health within the United Nations system.

Covid-19 vaccines from Pfizer, Moderna, and Astra Zeneca are very effective and safe. Two vaccines are required followed by a third booster vaccine after a period of time that, in view of the emergence of the Omicron strain of Covid, has been reduced to about three months as a result of declining antibody levels of protection. There is no doubt that vaccination has dramatically reduced the number of deaths and hospitalizations in the vaccinated population, leading to a decline in the prevalence of the diseases prevented. Unfortunately, those who resist vaccination fear the side effects that are considerably less than the complications and deaths that the primary disease is likely to cause and is grossly exaggerated on the Internet and sometimes by the media. There is now an active program for vaccinating schoolchildren who can contact Covid-19 infection that usually runs a milder course than that in an adult, but children can actively spread the disease to adults. A concern in children has been the development of myocarditis, an inflammatory disorder of cardiac muscle, but this has been shown to be much more common in people with the disease than in those who have been vaccinated against it. The resistance in the population of so many to receiving vaccination is a great concern particularly in countries where vaccination levels are low and the disease is spreading rapidly, causing increased hospitalization, dislocation of healthcare systems, and increased deaths from Covid. Omicron has also prevented people from being treated for other major killing disorders, the numbers of which are rising as a result of a lack of healthcare facilities in hospitals overcrowded with Covid sufferers. Vaccination has, however, undoubtedly been shown to be the best method of controlling the disease.

Despite the devastating effects of Covid-19 and the number of deaths now amounting to some five million, this remains less than the number of deaths that occur from the other diet-related killers described herein.

One of the major killers in the world is malaria caused by bites from infected female Anopheles mosquitoes. There are about 250 million cases per year with 500,000 deaths. Recently an effective vaccine for malaria has been developed.

Meningitis is a life-threatening infection of the outer layers of the brain. It can be caused by a number of bacteria, viruses, and fungi, the major one being meningococcal meningitis. Vaccination is now available against most of these potentially killing organisms.

Poliomyelitis a highly debilitating viral infection has largely been eradicated worldwide by vaccination, having previously killed up to half a million people per year and permanently disabled many more.

Pneumonia is an infection of the lungs that infects and kills almost a million children worldwide per year and affects all ages, particularly those over sixty-five years. Effective vaccination exists against the major bacterium pneumococcus.

Effective vaccination also exists against measles, mumps, pertussis, rubella, tetanus, and shingles.

Thus, vaccination has been a mass lifesaver over the last century preventing many millions of early deaths. Vaccination is safe, particularly so when the alternatives are considered. Vaccination against Covid-19 has represented a huge lifesaving advance and should be encouraged throughout the world so that ultimately virtually everyone receives it.

CHAPTER 16
SMOKING

It is fundamentally important to eliminate smoking, both active and passive, from our lives. This includes cigarettes, E-cigarettes, cigars, and pipes. In terms of your health, lungs, and potential longevity, it is undoubtedly the worst thing you can do, and every effort must be made to completely eliminate it from your life.

Currently 14 percent of United States adults aged eighteen or older smoke cigarettes. This means that an estimated 34.1 million people are regular smokers and more than sixteen million live with a smoking-related disease, coronary artery disease, vascular disease, heart failure, lung cancer, and other cancers. In the United States, smoking accounts for 480,000 deaths every year, or about one in five adults.

Regular smoking has, in fact, declined in the United States from 20.9 percent in 2005 to 14 percent in 2019. Men are more likely (15 percent) to smoke than women (12.7 percent). The prevalence is higher in younger people aged between twenty-five and forty-four years (16.7 percent) than in those between forty-five and sixty-four years (14 percent), and is lowest in those aged eighteen to twenty-four years (8.2 percent). According to the CDC, the groups of people with the highest incidence of smoking habit are men, those with lower educational achievements, those living below the poverty level, and those who live in the Midwest and southern states; the uninsured; the disabled; those with serious psychological issues; American Indians; Alaskan natives; and the LGBT group. Cigarettes are now very expensive.

With the quarantines imposed by the Covid outbreak Americans bought more cigarettes in 2020, the first increase in twenty years. The number of cigarettes purchased by wholesalers and retailers rose by 4 percent to a staggering 203.7 billion.

Smoking is highly addictive, and dependency often begins in the early years of life, causing progressive damage with aging, and is difficult for the individual to stop. Smokers are at higher risk of developing Covid-19 infection and because of underlying lung damage are more likely to develop complications and to die from the disease. Now that Covid is with us and is likely to stay, there is an even greater need for people to abandon cigarettes. Smoking causes cancer, heart disease, stroke, lung diseases, diabetes, and vascular disease. It also increases the risk for tuberculosis, certain infective diseases, and problems of the immune system, including rheumatoid arthritis, as a result of depressed immunity.

While smoking can suppress the appetite and contribute to weight loss, stopping smoking can lead to weight gain due to substituting sweets or snacks for tobacco, but this is no reason to smoke as the damages to your health from smoking greatly outweigh any possible slight advantage in terms of a small amount of weight loss.

Chapter 17
Nonalcoholic Fatty Disease of the Liver

Nonalcoholic fatty disease of the liver affects about a quarter of Americans. This is not related to alcohol but can be made worse by excess alcohol intake. It occurs when excess unhealthy ingested fat is stored in the liver, causing damage. In most the disease does not go on to become fatal, but in some it does progress to become a severe form of liver impairment that causes swelling and inflammation of the liver, leading to fibrosis or cirrhosis with ultimately liver failure and death. Those at risk are again the obese, particularly the morbidly obese, diabetics, those with high cholesterol and triglycerides, and those with hypertension—the same causes as pertain in all of the other major killers.

Signs of developing liver failure are swelling of the abdomen; itching; jaundice (i.e. yellow discoloration of the eyes and skin); spiderlike small vessels on the skin of the upper chest, face, and arms; a tremor of the hand; red discoloration of the palms; spontaneous bruising; Dupuytren's contracture; and mental impairment.

Drinking coffee has recently been shown to reduce liver disease by 21 percent, so drinkers are less likely to die from it. Also, it has been shown in three large studies that drinking coffee reduces heart failure and tea also can reduce the risk of Alzheimer's disease by 28 percent.

This, again, is a disease of dietary indiscretion, which in the early stages is potentially reversible by eating a healthy diet, exercising, losing weight, and avoiding excess alcohol intake.

Chapter 18
Illegal Drugs

The distribution and use of illegal drugs has escalated exponentially in recent years. These are largely imported through the Mexican border and distributed throughout the United States. The most commonly used drug is cannabis, which is now legal in some states even though it is potentially extremely damaging. More powerful drugs like heroin are now being focused on by dealers, which are highly addictive and very destructive.

Hundreds of drug dealers are using Instagram and the social media to market potent cannabis to children in a multi-billion dollar business. The problem on the Facebook-owned site has markedly increased over the lockdown leading to fears of the drug causing a "psychosis time bomb."

A drug baron known as "the Devil" has boasted about kidnapping and chopping off the fingers of child clients. This dealer has spread his business across to Great Britain using a social media site to earn themselves millions. These dealers have gathered almost 30,000 followers and advertise cannabis with enticing pictures of cannabis-packed attractive sweets and other edible materials, and they arrange for sales via private messaging services even reaching children in primary schools.

Many children taking these drugs develop heart palpitations, anxiety attacks, vomiting, paranoia, depression, and hallucinations. The high-strength cannabis trade has exploded during the lockdown and has driven many young people into psychosis and suicide. In the UK, it has been estimated that 8 percent of school pupils have used cannabis, leading to 13,000 requiring hospital treatment last year alone and more than 1000 being under the age of thirteen. Most sales are now being made online, which replaces street corner activity, and the market has been valued at between two and 2.6 billion pounds in the UK alone. Instagram makes it easier and safer for multiple dealers to expand their business. High potency cannabis now contains levels of up to 16 percent of THC, the psychoactive substance which has increased from 5 percent in the 1960s. Facebook, who owns Instagram, claims to have removed 2.3 million pieces of drug sales advertising content in a three-month period but still the business is rife and is growing increasing its harmful effects on health.

Chapter 19
Inflammatory Age

Scientists at Stanford University are claiming that rather than gaging the state of our health based upon increasing age in calendar years, we should be looking at the phenomenon of "inflammatory age." They have developed a blood test to measure chronic inflammation and state that it could provide an early warning of inflammation-related conditions, from which all of the major killers from heart disease to dementia could develop. This would give us an opportunity to take action to prevent the onset of these diseases as the changes are reversible. Dr. Sayed of Stanford University has reported in the Journal Nature Aging that inflammation is an important factor in the progression of the aging process. Chronic inflammation is a lingering, low level form of inflammation that can, over time, damage our cells and organs and is linked to all the major killing diseases, in particular type II diabetes and cancer.

Levels of inflammation increase with the aging process as a result of inflammatory molecules entering the body cells. It is exacerbated by factors such as obesity, diabetes, drug taking, atmospheric pollution, stress, and smoking. In terms of the progression of this underlying disease process, there is little to make us aware of its onset until we start to develop symptoms of which the first is often an increase in blood pressure.

These researchers have analyzed the levels of cytokines in the blood of over 1000 patients and have found these levels to be a more significant and appropriate indicator of generalized ill health than chronological age as a single factor alone. This gives an indication of biological age, which may be more important than chronological age, and the cytokine signature is an accurate indicator of overall body ill health. The researchers used these factors to calculate a person's realistic age rather than their chronological age, which correlated as an ultimate indicator of ill health based on the level of inflammation.

An example quoted is that if someone who is forty-five years old has an age indicated by the inflammatory parameters of sixty-five years, then the body is twenty years older than it should be due to the damaging effect of inflammation, and this is a better marker of their health than is their chronological age. We are all aware of how some people appear to age more rapidly than others of a similar chronological age. Their thesis is that inflammatory age is the major factor underlying the development of all of the major killing diseases.

Using blood samples, they calculated the inflammatory age of thirty-seven people from an area in Italy. Half of these participants were aged between fifty and seventy and were in excellent health for their age, and some individuals in this geographical area lived to be over 100 years old. The centenarians, on average had an inflammatory age forty years younger than their actual age. In contrast, most of the young group had an age that was higher than their chronological age. The authors quoted one super healthy 105-year-old man who astonishingly had a measured inflammatory age similar to that of a twenty-five-year-old. He was not frail and was capable of maintaining the normal day-to-day activities required in keeping a viable and healthy lifestyle. Furthermore, these investigators were able to identify those who developed heart failure years before this led to their early death.

The new test is several years away from widespread routine use and is probably valuable when used along with cholesterol, triglycerides, and C-reactive protein levels.

Those with a high inflammatory age assessment could reduce this by modifying their diet and exercising, both of which factors dampen chronic inflammation. Their research has shown that a cytokine called CXCL9 is strongly related to inflammatory age, suggesting that if a new drug could be specifically channeled against this, the effects in terms of being lifesaving could be phenomenal, helping life expectancy to significantly increase. It must be said, however, that aging is a multi-complex situation and there may be many hitherto undefined factors that could move the equation one way or another.

Chapter 20
Exercise

The importance of exercise cannot be overemphasized. Exercise is important from the point of view of preventing heart attacks, strokes, and the development of diabetes. The benefits of exercise are clearly visible by increased muscle mass, increased activity, and alertness. Exercise does not necessarily increase hunger. In fact, a thirty-to-forty-minute walk produces wellbeing by virtue of an endorphin drive and can lead to a suppression of appetite. Also, the results of participating in an exercise program are a disincentive for a person then to go home and eat excessive amounts of food. Exercise not only burns calories in itself but tends to increase basal metabolic rate for several hours, giving rise to a further erosion on the calorific load. Another useful manifestation of exercise is that it stimulates muscle production and converts fat into muscle. In addition, the endorphin drive produced by exercise results in a feeling of well-being and enables people to adopt a more positive attitude towards life and its problems.

The normal day-to-day relatively sedentary activities are between 500 and 1,000 calories of metabolic activity above the basal metabolic rate. Walking produces energy expenditure of 300 calories per hour. The body needs to burn 600 calories before it begins to burn fat. This would mean walking for two hours or a distance of approximately six miles a day. Doubling that to four hours or twelve miles a day would, on that day, burn 82 grams of fat, about one fifth of a pound. Cycling will typically burn about 400 calories per hour, running between 500 and 600 calories, rowing, and swimming between 500 and 600 calories per hour. While increasing numbers of people run marathons, greater numbers refrain from indulging in any form of physical activity at all. Physical energy expenditure ranges from static physical exercise, such as rapidly increasing and decreasing muscle tone and gesticulating, to voluntarily moving in athletic activity such as running.

Whatever your age, attending a gymnasium is good. All forms of physical activity contribute to maintaining good bodily and mental health. Working with weights burns calories and increases muscle. Cycling and swimming are excellent forms of exercise. Participating in classes such as body tone, body conditioning, HIIT, and Pilates in the gymnasium is good. These activities involve supervised group sessions that produce more controlled activity and a good psychological affect.

Many of the killing conditions are more likely attributed to low physical activity and cardiorespiratory fitness than obesity per se. Exercise protects the blood vessels by giving them a workout. This helps control blood pressure and provides oxygenation to tissues. Aerobic exercise is good because it raises the heart rate and stimulates breathing, and hence the oxygenation of cells. Healthy exercise includes all activities such as brisk walking, swimming, jogging, or playing tennis. It also helps to maintain normal blood sugar levels and increase good HDL cholesterol. All of these factors protect against the major killers. Walking is a good exercise particularly brisk walking. Ideally attempt to do more than 5000 steps per day, which is at least two miles, or if you have time try to get in 10,000 steps daily.

The effects of physical exercise in relation to total energy turnover each day are, on the whole, relatively small. It has been shown that those who walk more, however, weigh less. Furthermore, the decline in physical activity in the population as a whole probably contributes to the increased prevalence of obesity. The exact mechanism of this is not fully understood. It is possible that the decrease in activity that occurs with increasing age may form the basis for the decline in muscle mass and lean body mass as people grow older. Replacement of lean tissue by fat associated with aging worsens the problem of energy imbalance since the basal need for energy falls with the total reduction in metabolically active lean tissue. This will lead to a further drop in the basal metabolic rate and a tendency to gain body fat. It should be emphasized that the physiological beneficial effects of short periods of moderately intense exercise are well-documented, and that the minimum of twenty minutes of moderate activity three times per week is good for the cardiovascular system. This degree of activity also seems to play an important role in improving an individual's sense of wellbeing, probably by the production of endorphins. It is unclear whether this amount of exercise helps to maintain lean body mass. Not only are the effects of an aerobic exercise positive, but exercise is good for the brain.

Lack of exercise is an important factor in the obesity equation. It has been shown that the less walking a person does in his day-to-day activities, the more likely he is to be overweight. Exercise increases academic performance, assertiveness, confidence, emotional stability, independence, memory, mood, sexual satisfaction, and well-being. In addition, exercise programs decrease absenteeism, anger, anxiety, depression, and even alcohol abuse. Obese subjects are often opposed to exercise programs. They are self-conscious and frequently have difficulty in performing the exercises because they are carrying so much extra weight, or they may be restricted by joint pains or breathlessness. Many morbidly obese subjects are too disabled to exercise or even to climb a flight of stairs. Those who can exercise are frequently discouraged by the slow results achieved from exercise programs and the fact that a can of cola contains all the calories expended in a thirty-minute exercise schedule.

Exercising for fifteen to twenty-five minutes a day can extend your life expectancy by up to three years if you are obese, and seven years if you are in good shape. Brisk walking improves cardiovascular health and reduces diabetes and hypertension. It can also improve anxiety and depression but doesn't usually result in any weight loss if it is confined to such a short period of activity.

There has been a long-standing and hitherto unanswered question as to whether exercise makes us eat more afterwards or decreases our appetite for the next meal. A recent study investigated physically inactive males and females and found that those who worked out when given a lunch afterwards did not overeat, but they didn't skip dessert or take small portions afterwards. Fewer calories are burned by exercise than eating at a standard restaurant meal, 300 calories for one hour's walking versus 1000 calories for the restaurant meal. This suggests that exercise itself will not tend to make us eat less or lose weight, but it is a valuable component in our overall healthcare strategy.

A number of studies have shown that those who begin an exercise program do not want to decrease as much weight as the alleged calories burnt actually suggest, mainly because our bodies are wired through the years of evolution to hold onto fat stores as a way to protect us from famine, which has been the major nutritional problem for tens of thousands of years leading up to the last century. Some studies suggested that very strenuous exercise, which is prolonged, decreased people's appetite for hours into the following day, while, in contrast, other studies found people eating more at their next meal after working out, so the question remains unresolved.

In the initial studies, the patients aged between eighteen and fifty-five were overweight and did not, prior to the study, do much exercise. The subjects who participated visited the lab every morning for breakfast and then walked at a brisk pace for forty-five minutes. Afterwards, they were given an appetizing buffet lunch, complete with salad, soda, lasagna, and pound cake. The results showed that the volunteers not only did not feel more or less hungry after their workouts compared with the just sitting participants, but they also ate about the same amount during lunch regardless of whether they were working out or not. The study suggests that the above brisk walking or weightlifting does not influence eating habits despite them being given an appetizing large meal. This study, however, has limitations because it has only examined at one session of moderate exercise a small number of patients who were out of shape. It is possible that a different cross-section of the community with different underlying health issues behave differently. The study concluded that exercise might help with weight control, noting that the essence of the study was that exercise only burned 300 calories per hour compared to 1000 calories in the test meal. Having said that, I do believe that exercise is important in maintaining optimal health. There are some reservations to this study that presents an unrepresentative cross-section of the community, small numbers of participants, and a short term of study.

Chapter 21
Sleep

Sleep is as vital to our physical and mental well-being as food and water. Without enough of it we become unable to operate properly, and our cognitive function can markedly decline. Studies on millions of people have shown that less sleep can lead to a shorter life. Less sleep results in hypertension, obesity, heart disease, diabetes, Alzheimer's disease, and impaired immune functioning—in fact, all of the major killers discussed herein. Interrupted sleep patterns have been used in interrogation methods on prisoners. Chronic insomnia affects about 10 percent of adults and 30 percent have interrupted sleep on an intermittent basis. It is recommended that one should aim to have seven hours of sleep per night. We spend one third of our lives sleeping, but is it important to health?

The Covid crisis has greatly increased people's problems with sleeping, which develop in 75 percent of those suffering from the virus. This may be due to damage to the nervous system. It is particularly true in people with long Covid and can result from the isolation caused by lockdowns. Those who are sleep deprived are more likely to succumb to the virus.

Fifty percent of people with insomnia have a mental health diagnosis such as depression or anxiety. Sleep deprivation is associated with higher levels of cortisol and adrenaline, which affect the heart and blood vessels. This only occurs in those whose sleep is severely curtailed to less than five hours per night, and in these emotional consequences develop such as low mood, anxiety, and irritability.

As we age our circadian sleep cycles shorten and many become sleepless in old age, but super agers sleep for at least eight hours a night. A nap in the daytime also helps to relieve stress. During sleep toxins are cleared from the brain and cells repair and regrow. A buildup of toxins in the brain leads to inflammation that can destroy blood vessels and interfere with cellular function. Sleep improves cellular mechanisms and can improve memory, particularly short-term memory, which tends to be compromised by aging. Impaired sleep patterns occur with the early symptoms of dementia and increase as the disease progresses. Removal of toxins from the brain during sleep may prevent the buildup of amyloid plaques that destroy brain cells in Alzheimer's disease. Interrupted sleep patterns that occur with sleep apnea, anxiety, and depression are associated with a higher risk of dementia. Sleeping less at night seems to affect the hormonal patterns that regulate hunger and satiety leading to obesity, sleep apnea, and a higher incidence of dementia.

Throughout life seven to nine hours of sleep at night seems optimal. Deep sleep and restorative slow wave sleep patterns tend to reduce with age. Sleep can also be interrupted by painful conditions such as joint and back disease, and there is a higher incidence of gastroesophageal reflux disease, which is exacerbated by eating shortly before retiring.

A regular sleep rhythm is good. Eating a heavy meal or intense exercise should be avoided late at night, as these stimulate the metabolism and increase awareness. The bedroom should be dark and silent. Today, so many are using social media, reading emails, and looking at phones throughout the night, which are clearly obstructing normal sleep.

A recent study of 88,000 people published in the European Heart Journal found that those who went to sleep between 10:00 p.m. and 11:00 p.m. had a lower risk of cardiovascular disease and stroke than those who had a shorter sleep period. The reasons suggested for this is that 82 percent of the population is genetically programmed to fall asleep at about this time and to wake up seven or eight hours later. This is the case in order to stay healthy and to synchronize sleeping habits with built-in circadian rhythms. It has been shown that an adequate period of duration of sleep improves mental health. If we go to bed much earlier or later, it interferes with our circadian rhythm leading to more disturbed sleep. This was suggested to explain the 24 percent spike in heart attacks that occurs in association with Daylight Savings Time on the day after the change, which disturbs our body clock. Disturbed sleep increases the risk of heart attacks in part because it leads to a rise in blood pressure. Sleep activates relaxation, growth, repair, recovery, and immunity. When sleep is disturbed the hormones cortisol and adrenaline rapidly increase, and this increases the wear and tear on blood vessels, in particular the coronary arteries. It also effects insulin release and sensitivity producing a prediabetic state. Sleep also plays a part in cleaning up the arteries and reducing plaque deposits. It is essential to wind down, relax, and avoid a large meal or a lot of alcohol before going to bed. A walk early in the morning is a good way of activating healthy body function early in the day.

It is common and not abnormal to wake up several times at night, and this is best coped with by continuing to rest in bed, as you will fall asleep again. Coffee, which has a half-life of about six hours, should not be drunk after midday. It is a stimulant that can be helpful in the mornings but later interferes with sleep. People who exercise regularly fall asleep sooner though they do not sleep for longer periods of time.

Poor sleep habits are linked to bad snack choices throughout the day, according to a study from Ohio State University. Data from 20,000 people were reviewed relating to their eating habits and to sleep. Those who slept less consumed more calories, carbohydrates, sugar, and caffeine. The study concluded that the longer we are awake the more we eat and we tend to eat the wrong things, which ultimately can be life-threatening.

Studies have shown that less than six hours of sleep daily can adversely affect brain health, increase the risk of Alzheimer's disease, increase heart problems, and reduce life expectancy. A healthy sleep routine is essential to keep the immune system optimally functioning and effective in fighting off illnesses such as influenza and viral infections. Early morning wakening, typically at about 3:00 a.m., and not getting back to sleep is a common problem affecting all ages and has been named "mornsomnia."

Throughout the day the brain produces toxins the accumulation of which is associated with neurocognitive decline leading to Alzheimer's disease. When we sleep, production of toxins stops and cerebral fluid is produced, which clears the brain of these accumulated toxins. During sleep increased immunity is manifest by a buildup of cytokines that target infection and inflammation. Those who are sleep deprived have more than a twofold greater risk of colds and flu. Adequate sleep helps how we respond to vaccines by increasing antibody production. A power nap of twenty minutes can be good and can improve alertness during the day.

Sleeping pills can certainly work but should be avoided if at all possible. Benzodiazepines are the most commonly prescribed drugs and increasing doses are frequently given, which can lead to dependency. They also impair memory and can reduce alertness and mental capacity the following day. Melatonin, the sleep hormone taken in tablet form, is widely used, since natural levels become depleted with age. It can be helpful particularly in the elderly, but I do not encourage its use. There are many over-the-counter herbal remedies such as valerian and passionflower but, on the whole, these are of little value.

It is important to establish regular sleeping times, restrict light exposure in the bedroom, and not eat or drink coffee late at night. Set a wake-up time seven to eight hours later. Daily exercise is helpful for a healthy sleep pattern and tends to reduce anxiety. If possible, it should be carried out outside in daylight. Stop consuming caffeine at lunch time. Alcohol can induce sleep, but it is a stimulant, so drinking at night tends to lead to disrupted sleep patterns. Nicotine is also a stimulant, it goes without saying, so don't smoke. Try to avoid stressful activities or worrying aspects of life late at night. This will produce anxiety and prevent sleep induction.

Sleep, therefore, is part of the equation in maintaining a long and healthy life. It isn't just important for replenishing energy levels. Scientists increasingly believe it affects brain function in the long term and influences the risk of dementia and Parkinson's disease.

CHAPTER 22
FURTHER PSYCHOLOGICAL FACTORS

Psychological factors are commonly associated with weight gain. This can also relate to modern-day lifestyle; for example, working from home during the Covid crisis led to a high incidence of weight gain.

Social isolation when working from home becomes a manifestation of the obese state and produces depression and food provides solace to the depressed producing further weight gain. All of the major killers can lead to mental changes. The massively increased prevalence of the major killers and of obesity in the last half century cannot be attributed to either a change in genetics or the incidence of recognizable psychiatric disorders. It is rather clearly behavioral, cultural, and a submission to extrinsic pressures, such as food advertisements, and a consequence of acquired aberration of the role and value of nutrients. Such behavioral influences may have led more people to "live to eat" rather than "eat to live." This would suggest addictive behavior, of which there may clearly be a component. Addiction to food is ostensibly more of a problem than addiction to alcohol or drugs because, difficult as the latter two are to manage, the patient may temporally be taken away from alcohol or drugs whilst food is always essential. Not only is food essential—"We are what we eat"—it's accurate balance, as a health provider, may clearly be extremely difficult to control once the homeostatic mechanisms fall away.

The homeostatic mechanisms that regulate eating behavior, present throughout the animal kingdom, are becoming grossly distorted in man for the first time in thousands of years. Throughout history, man has clearly suffered more from the ravages of starvation than from a plethora of food, but gluttony and obesity existed with other excesses in the period of affluence of the Roman area. Although the ravages of malnutrition and the extremes of starvation in Nigeria and other African countries are depicted periodically by the media, we appear now to have, again, entered an era where more suffer from excess of rather than the shortage of food. A remarkable degree of sophistication and control goes into body weight maintenance. The twenty-pound weight gain experienced by the average American between the ages of twenty-five and fifty-five represents a remarkably small net imbalance between energy intake and expenditure—an excess of intake over expenditure of 0.3 percent of ingested calories or approximately six calories per day!

The eating of food has become an important ritual. We all like good foods, a variety of foods, and we not only socialize around the table, but we hold business meetings around it as well. If indeed food becomes an addiction, which is the case in some morbidly obese individuals, then it is one with which the addicted must constantly contend, as food is not only essential but is around us always.

Diets eaten in different countries vary very widely, but most nations have, over the centuries, developed diets, which, though widely differing in their content, maintain the body in good functional health without any marked nutritional deficiencies. Recently studies have shown that the longer Puerto Rican women live in the continental United States and improve their knowledge of English, the more their weight increases. This is persuasive evidence that social factors, rather than genetic ones, are important. It is also true that immigrants from different parts of the world in the second generation develop the same pattern of diseases as are prevalent in the country to which they have migrated.

Numerous biological and psychological influences may modify eating behavior. Dietary composition per se is not an exact determinant of body makeup. It is the total caloric intake that is the major factor. As both protein and carbohydrates can efficiently be converted into fat, there is no evidence that changing the relative proportions of protein, carbohydrate, and fat in the diet without reducing overall caloric intake will promote significant weight loss.

Though perhaps difficult accurately to categorize, the psychological factors that pertain to an obese state are significant and considerable. The higher the body mass index, the greater is the incidence of depression. A number of factors contribute to the development of psychological problems that culminate in chronic depression. Discrimination, which occurs towards the obese, leads to low self-worth and a reduced quality of life. Family and sexual relationships suffer, and problems frequently arise in the workplace.

Body image is an aspect of overall self-image. A woman who was sexually abused in childhood may use her size as protection against attracting men. Despite her desire to lose weight, she may get more and more anxious as she becomes more shapely. Another person who equates food with love or weight with power will experience such inner conflict about changing his or her lifestyle when losing weight.

Early in the twentieth century, when tuberculosis and other infectious diseases were still rampant, to be thin was often perceived as a sign of sickness, poverty, or neglect. The prime of families in those days was plump, healthy children; the plump female was womanly, the plump male, with watch chain stretched across his belly, looked prosperous. Most people had heard of calories and knew that sweets were fattening, but paid little or no attention to the caloric contents of what they ate. In marked contrast, after the 1960s, the attractive female body image became one of increasing thinness even amounting to anorexia.

To be successful all psychotherapy must address emotional dysregulation, impulsive behavior, and cognitive and perceptual distortions. Group and individual therapy, particularly cognitive behavioral therapy, can highlight rationalizations, reframe negative patterns of thinking, and provide a more realistic manner of self-assessment. A recognition of one's own mental functioning and how one solves problems is essential to reshape these attitudes from the past, which may sabotage dieting efforts.

After World War II, the biggest change in American life came with the availability of television sets. These changed the eating habits of America, but not for the better. The TV dinner predominated on the American menu as everyone gathered around the new center of the home. Television's advertising potential was quickly realized and exploited by the food industry, tempting adults to indulge in double cheeseburgers, chips, and multiple snacks.

Advertising showed America the picture of affluence and the carefree existence untouched by war or want. Cars became oversized, sporting huge fins and capacious cross bench seats. Supermarkets replaced the corner shops selling countless food packages. As a consequence, people began progressively to overeat, culminating in the crisis of today.

PART 2

Chapter 23
How to Modify a Poor Diet

In part one of this book, all of today's major killers have been outlined:

- coronary artery disease
- heart failure
- cardiac arrhythmias
- arteriosclerosis
- prediabetes
- diabetes
- vascular disease
- cancer
- dementia
- liver disease
- joint disease

Obesity in isolation can be the major factor in all of these, and there is a single underlying cause in every one of these killers: an unhealthy, abnormal diet in the long term.

Let us now analyze the causative factors in diet and how to control or modify these. Your moments of deepest concentration should be focused on your life. It is in your hands, and you are in control. In order to control the causative issues, there are simple rules outlined here that can lead you into optimizing the quality of your existence, your overall health, and its probable duration. Here is what you have to do.

The questions we need to address are:

1. Which foods are damaging?
2. How can we control calorie intake?
3. What are the basic principles of nutrition?
4. What are the major sources of energy required for nutritionally a healthy body?
5. What do we need to do about vitamins and minerals?
6. How do we need to convert energy intake along with eating healthily?
7. What is the most healthy and economically viable weight-reducing diet?
8. What should we do about optimizing exercise?
9. How important is stress and its control in the equation?
10. Are there any medications which we could use prophylactically?
11. How much time should we spend sleeping?
12. How much alcohol is it safe to drink?

Let's address these issues and see how our lifestyle and longevity can potentially be improved and let's do it the easy way.

The foods most damaging to our health are principally refined carbohydrates and, to a lesser extent, trans fatty acids.

Refined carbohydrates cause the blood sugar to rise rapidly, and these are the main enemy. Not all carbohydrates are bad. Many vegetables and fruits are high in vitamins and minerals. They also contain antioxidants that dispose of the potentially harmful oxygen byproducts called oxygen free radicals. Vegetables also contain fiber, which can lower cholesterol and stabilize blood sugar levels. Therefore, the best advice is to recommend a strategy of eating in moderation and avoiding refined carbohydrates and trans fats. Eat minimally processed foods, for example, brown rice rather than white rice, blueberries, and other berries. Fish, garlic, and olive oil are also good components of the diet.

When preparing meats for cooking, external fat should be removed. Portions should be restricted to the size of the palm of the hand. Expensive cuts of beef taste better because they contain more fat. It is much better to eat lean meat and to reduce the amount of red meat taken to a maximum of one meal per week. Veal is low in fat but high in cholesterol. Lamb and pork tend to contain a lot of fat. Cutting the fat from pork leaves healthy, lean meat. Bacon is high in sodium and in fat, and sausages are high in refined carbohydrates and fat. Chicken is high in protein and low in fat and cholesterol. Chicken without the skin makes for healthy eating. Turkey is the leanest meat of all and with the skin removed the fat content of turkey breast is less than 1 percent. Contrary to popular belief, duck, with the skin removed, is low in fat. Game birds such as pheasant are very low in fat. Wild game like deer are a good source of protein and also low in fat. Always remove the skin from chicken, turkey, duck, and pheasant and these will then provide food that is low in fat and high in protein with an exclusion of the cholesterol. Milk contains calcium, protein, zinc, and the fat-soluble vitamins. Cheese is similar to milk but more concentrated. Egg yolks are high in cholesterol though the whites are an excellent source of protein, and the yolks are not necessarily bad because an egg only contains about seventy calories. Yogurt is acceptable but tends to be sweetened with refined sugar, which is usually indicated on the label, and those with added sugar should be avoided. The classical English breakfast of bacon, eggs, and sausage fried in butter is not a healthy start to the day. Margarines are free of trans fats and contain twice as much polyunsaturated as saturated fat, so they are a more healthy source of fat than pure butter. Vegetable oils, particularly olive oil, are good, as they contain large amounts of heart healthy omega-3 and omega-6 fatty acids.

Nuts contain a large amount of fat but also many beneficial nutrients such as B vitamins. They are good in small amounts. Coconuts are high in phytosterols, compounds that have been shown to reduce the levels of cholesterol in the blood. They are, however, also high in saturated fats and carbohydrates but contain no cholesterol. Vital nutrients are plentiful in seeds, which also contain fiber and omega-3 fatty acids. Flax seeds are particularly high in omega-3 fatty acids and have anticoagulant properties. They are an excellent source of nutrition, and it has been suggested that they may be beneficial in preventing the development of some tumors.

Soy protein is the only complete vegetable protein that contains all of the essential amino acids. Soy also contains iron, calcium, magnesium, vitamin D, riboflavin, thiamine, folate, and good fats. Soy flour is higher in protein and lower in carbohydrates than wheat flour. Legumes are low in fat and contain no cholesterol. They are rich in minerals and fiber. Humus contains a high concentration of fat.

Bread is high in calories and carbohydrates. Croissants are the most calorie dense. A bagel can contain 400 calories, which does not provide a good nutrition to calorie intake ratio. Whole wheat bread is the lowest in calories, at 45 calories per slice and the highest in fiber. There are a wide variety of these available and they provide the best source of more healthy nutrition from bread products. Muffins need not be so calorie dense, but they do contain trans fatty acids. Pasta is low in fat and cholesterol but high in carbohydrates. White rice is rich in refined carbohydrates, low in fat and cholesterol, but also contains a good source of B vitamins. Whole grains are digested slowly, and therefore, they don't produce rapid rises in blood glucose levels, which predisposes a person to diabetes. Most cereals are a rich source of carbohydrates and although other nutrients may be added, breakfast cereals should not be part of the diet. Of all the cereals grains and grasses, oats are the most nutritious. They provide more protein than rice and they contain multiple vitamins, iron, selenium, and fiber.

Fruits and vegetables are most important in a healthy diet. They are rich in antioxidants and contain vitamins, minerals, and fiber. Highest in antioxidants are blueberries, and blue, red, and purple berries are high in anthocyanins. The healthiest of all vegetables is asparagus. Broccoli is also a very healthy source of nutrition. Carrots are rich in vitamin A but contain a little more carbohydrate than most vegetables. Onions and garlic are an excellent source of food and are also helpful in preventing thrombosis in vessels as they have a mild anticoagulant content. Fruits are a good source of energy but on the whole vegetables are better than fruits, though don't dismiss the latter if you are hungry between meals as they are much more beneficial than the alternative cakes and biscuits as snacks. On the whole try not to eat snacks. Some of us have food cravings particularly for sweet foods like cakes or chocolate. Most cravings are psychological and when you eat sweets your body releases the chemical serotonin in your brain, which gives a feeling of well-being. These sort of cravings for snacks produce a rapid elevation of blood glucose, which in turn causes increased insulin concentration sending the blood glucose down sometimes to a low level creating further hunger, which makes the craving return, and more calories are ingested from the sweets you crave. A 100-gram block of chocolate contains about 500 calories.

Probably the biggest contemporary problem that affects so many of us in relation to obesity is the social trend, or compulsion, to eat in fast food restaurants or do takeouts. A single meal of a super burger, jumbo fries, mega soda, and fried pie greatly exceeds the total daily recommended caloric intake and is high in sodium but deficient in vitamins and minerals. Just the beef part of a double burger contains 518 calories with 33 grams of fat and 47 grams of carbohydrates. Whether purchased from McDonald's or Burger King, the calorific counts are similar. Kentucky Fried Chicken contains a large amount of fat in the batter and in the skin of the chicken. An extra crispy breast contains 470 calories, and a chunky chicken pot pie exceeds 770 calories. Most main courses of meals served in fast food restaurants contain in excess of 1000 calories. Taco Bell's products tend to be lower in cholesterol, but the taco salad with a fried tortilla shell contains a staggering 800 calories. This makes a taco salad higher in saturated fat, calories, carbohydrates, and sodium than a Big Mac or a Whopper. It is best to avoid pastries, toast, and white bread with your meals. One slice of a beef personal pan at Pizza Hut contains 710 calories. Pizzas are high in calories and whole pizzas can easily exceed 1200 calories. The thicker the crust, the more calories and the more unhealthy the pizza is, so pizzas do not create a healthy form of eating.

Eating out in restaurants continues to be increasingly popular. The pressures of modern economics in the family have led to both parents working full time, and when they return in the evening, they don't like cooking dinner. When visiting a restaurant, a buffet meal should be avoided. There is a great tendency to go back for second and third courses, and you have no idea of how many calories you are consuming. Restaurant portions tend to be large because the cost of providing food in a restaurant is the least of the overheads; most of the costs are consumed in paying rents and staff salaries. Desserts in restaurants always look attractive but are high in calories and full of sugar and should be avoided, if possible. Many restaurants today print the number of calories contained in most of the dishes on the menu, which is an excellent practice. When visiting the restaurant keep bread off the table. It is usual to eat a large amount of bread, often with butter, while waiting for the order to be delivered. It is also a good plan to take home half of your main course, which can provide you with another full meal the following day. Ordering a salad is sensible but avoid adding large amounts of mayonnaise or sweet dressings. Some available dressings are totally calorie free, such as honey mustard. If ordering wine, do so by the glass and have a medium-sized glass of about 150 milliliters, and try to stay with one glass rather than ordering it by the bottle. A bottle of wine has a volume of 750 milliliters with an alcohol content of about 14 percent, in addition to a considerable carbohydrate content in the sweeter wines. This gives a calorie content of 1050 calories without including the sugar, more than the main course in a fast-food restaurant. Not all vegetarian meals are low in calories; many exceed 1000 calories. Remember that the portions on your plate are about twice the amount you should eat. Portion sizes in restaurants have steadily increased in size since the end of World War II. Eating large steaks in steakhouses is unhealthy.

CHAPTER 24
NUTRITION AND METABOLISM

We derive all of our energy from three sources: proteins, carbohydrates, and fats. Proteins and carbohydrates provide four calories per gram; fat, nine calories per gram; and alcohol, eight calories per gram. One pound of butter provides 4000 calories; one pound of turkey breast, 1800 calories; and one pound of sugar, 1800 calories. With regard to alcohol, a one-liter bottle of whiskey, gin, vodka, or rum provides 3200 calories. So, avoid too much butter, don't drink too much, and make sure you get an adequate protein intake.

Under resting conditions, a normal healthy adult male burns approximately ten calories per pound of his body weight per day. With normal activity this calorie requirement virtually doubles. The basic requirement of living cells is to use protein for repair and replacement of cells and to supply energy to drive these reactions.

PROTEINS

Proteins provide the structure of cells in all living organisms. They are large molecules with high molecular weight, made up by junctions between numerous amino acids. These are the building units. The molecules are made up of carbon, oxygen, hydrogen, nitrogen, with in addition, in some, sulfur. The proteins contain the essential amino acids that make up DNA and RNA. They are essential for growth and maintenance and constantly turn over. Protein is required for growth and the maintenance of healthy tissue and protein needs are dependent upon your health and activity level.

Enzymes that enhance chemical reactions are made up of proteins, which are required for digestion, energy production, blood clotting, and muscle contraction. An adequate amount of protein intake is essential for body function and avoidance of illness. It stimulates the immune system. Antibodies consist of proteins that fight off viruses and bacteria. Hormones are made up of proteins such as insulin and glucagon. Proteins are required to make up the body strength and elasticity and also play a vital role in maintaining the correct balance between acids and bases in the body and maintain adequate fluid balance. Inadequate intake of protein results in fluid leaving the cells causing swelling or edema in the abdomen and around the ankles. Although protein in the body can be an energy source, it is only used in situations of fasting, exhaustive exercise, or inadequate calorie intake.

Essential good protein energizes and probably helps to lose weight. But protein, as in red meat, is toxic, predisposes you to heart disease, stroke, and cancer, and increases mortality at any age by about 20 percent. Some meats, however, are healthier than some vegetables. Protein is undoubtedly superior to low molecular weight carbohydrates and some fats. It makes you feel full earlier and more in a position to burn extra calories. Protein also, as stated, strengthens bones and improves muscle. Red meat, however, produces heart disease, diabetes, and cancer, and one hot dog per day increases mortality by 20 percent, two strips of bacon, likewise, and they increase the incidence of diabetes by 50 percent.

It has been shown in a number of studies that growth hormone promotes strength and muscle growth but increases the risk of cancer. A high protein diet with increasing growth hormone increases the death rate and these factors are a major cause of mortality. High levels of growth hormone increase the incidence of colon cancer. Bodybuilders who take growth hormone supplements have been estimated to being 34 percent more likely to die prematurely than people of the same age. You should reduce your eating of red meat to no more than twice per week. A Harvard study has shown that reducing the intake of red meat reduces heart disease, diabetes, and cancer by at least 14 percent. One of the problems of eating the healthy proteins is the use of antibiotics in chicken food to increase their growth rate. Wild fresh fish, particularly salmon, are a good additive to the diet but are expensive, but farm-raised salmon increases growth hormone and also serum levels of mercury. Protein present in vegetables can increase the immune response and is free from bad effects. In addition, it does not stimulate growth hormone production; therefore, ideally one should exchange red meat for eating healthy vegetables at least four times per week. Not all plants are healthy; lectins in some of them are not good. Lectins can lead to leaking from the gut with increased bloating and fatigue; therefore, too many lectins should be avoided. The really good vegetables from this aspect are spinach, broccoli, avocados, and Brussels sprouts. Flaxseed, spirulina, and hemp seed are also calorie free and good for weight loss. Electing to take a full diet based on plants, however, is not easy to access. Hemp seed is rich in omega-3 fatty acids and good for weight control and brain function. Whey protein that comes from cows' milk is high in lectins and is not good.

CARBOHYDRATES

Carbohydrates in the food can be enticing and comforting. They are, however, the real enemy underlying obesity, and simple carbohydrates are the harmful ones. Sticking to a low carbohydrate diet can be very difficult and usually in the long-term leads to failure.

Simple carbohydrates are rapidly absorbed in the intestine and are small molecules made up of one or two simple sugars, glucose, fructose, sucrose, or lactose. Candy, soda, syrups, cookies, pastries, and pasta are made up of simple carbohydrates. They have little or no nutritional value and tend to cause spikes in blood sugar.

Complex carbohydrates contain simple sugars conjoined to produce bigger molecules. These are digested and absorbed more slowly. Beans, peas, lentils, peanuts, potatoes, corn, cereals, and wholemeal bread are made up of complex carbohydrates. They make you feel full more quickly and stay full longer. They provide sustained energy but can still result in a high carbohydrate meal.

Bad carbohydrates cause obesity. They are low in fiber and high in calories and they metabolize rapidly causing spikes of blood sugar. They are white flour, pasta, mashed potatoes, and are often combined with fats such as butter, cholesterol, and trans fats. Good carbohydrates are complex carbohydrates. They are low in sodium but are large molecules that are more slowly absorbed and are not directly connected with heart conditions, diabetes, or obesity.

There is evidence that carbohydrates can be important in maintaining mental health and memory. Choosing the right complex carbohydrates for your diet can be helpful in stabilizing weight, while remembering to minimize simple carbohydrates. Foods high in carbohydrates are bread, cereal, pasta, white rice, cookies and cakes, sugary beverages, and potatoes. Oats are 70 percent carbohydrates, 15 percent fat, and 15 percent protein but also contain a lot of fiber so they are the best if you are taking a breakfast cereal. A banana contains 27 grams of carbohydrates, and they are high in bad carbohydrates. Plums are full of simple sugars. Good sources are lemons, broccoli, salmon, spinach, beans, nuts, avocados, onions, garlic, and berries—strawberries, raspberries, blackberries, and blueberries. Blueberries are the best because they have a unique level of antioxidants and overall are the best addition you can make to your diet, particularly for breakfast.

Fats

We need some fat in the diet but too much can raise your cholesterol and triglyceride levels increasing your risk of heart disease, stroke, hypertension, and liver failure. The body requires the ingestion of certain fatty acids. Fat helps the body absorb the essential vitamins A, D, and E, which are fat soluble. The main types of fat in food are saturated and unsaturated. Most fats and oils contain some of each of these but in different proportions. Saturated fats are bad, and their intake should be minimized. Foods containing large amounts of saturated fat are red meat, sausages, butter, cheese, cream, cookies, cakes, and pastries.

Cholesterol is a fatty substance ingested and manufactured in the liver. It is carried in the bloodstream as low-density lipoprotein's LDL and high-density lipoprotein's HDL. LDL is bad fat, which accelerates heart disease and the other major killers; HDL is good cholesterol, which takes cholesterol from the tissues and clears it in the liver.

The worst fats are trans fats found in red meats and dairy products. On the whole the normal diet contains much less trans fat than saturated fats. Monounsaturated fats are the best and are found in olive oil, avocados, and nuts. There are two types of polyunsaturated fats, omega-3 and omega-6. Omega-3 fats are found in high quantities in fish, salmon, trout, herring, mackerel. Omega-6 fats are found in vegetable oils, corn and sunflower. Eating fish is an excellent component to the diet. Fat is extracted from some supermarket products labeled "reduced fat," but they may still contain a considerable amount of fat.

Vitamins and Minerals

Many of the normal chemical processes in the body require vitamins. Deficiencies of these vitamins cause well-defined distinctive diseases. A total of thirteen vitamins have been identified as being essential in normal nutrition. Vitamins A, D, E, and K are fat soluble; B and C are water-soluble. The properties of these vitamins are briefly described below.

Vitamin A helps the body's natural defense against illness and infection. It can improve vision in dim light, and it helps to keep the skin healthy. Good sources of vitamin A are cheese, eggs, oily fish, milk, liver, and vegetables. You should be able to get all the vitamin A you need from your diet.

Vitamin B exists in a number of different forms. Vitamin B1, thiamine, is found in peas, fresh fruits, and whole grain breads. The body does not store it, but you should get enough on a daily basis from your diet. Vitamin B2, riboflavin, helps keep the skin, eyes, and nervous system healthy. Good sources are milk, eggs, and mushrooms. Adequate amounts are provided with a normal diet. Vitamin B3, niacin, is found in meat, fish, and eggs. Again, the normal diet provides enough to protect the nervous system and skin. Pantothenic acid is found in chicken, beef, eggs, mushrooms, and avocados. Vitamin B6, pyridoxine, helps the body to use and store energy and maintains the health of blood. It is found in meat, milk, and vegetables. Vitamin B7, biotin, is found in a wide range of foods, and it has been suggested that it stimulates hair growth. Folic acid is a very important vitamin essential for maintaining healthy red cells in the blood and reducing the incidence of spina bifida in unborn babies. It is found in largest amounts in green vegetables. Vitamin B-12 is essential for maintaining healthy red blood cells and an intact nervous system. It is found in meat, milk, and eggs. Living on a vegan diet can produce deficiencies with damage to the nervous system.

Vitamin C, ascorbic acid, is essential in maintaining healthy skin, gums, blood vessels, bone, and cartilage. Deficiency causes scurvy that used to be common on long sea voyages and became treatable by the provision of limes to sailors who became known as limeys. Mixed vegetables are a good source of vitamin C.

Vitamin D helps regulate the amount of calcium in bone. Exposure to sunlight provides most of the vitamin D we require. It has been reported that it may be helpful in preventing and treating Covid 19.

Vitamin E is found in a wide variety of foods and helps maintain healthy skin and eyes and strength of the body's immune system.

Vitamin K is essential for normal blood clotting and helping wounds to heal. It is found in green vegetables.

Antioxidants are substances that slow or prevent the oxidation of other substances. Oxidation produces oxygen free radicals, substances that damage cells. Antioxidants have been widely used in dietary supplements with the intention of preventing heart disease and cancer. Clinical trials, however, have not proven or established benefits of antioxidant supplements. Sources of food rich in antioxidants are fruits, vegetables, whole grains, and olive oil.

Minerals

In addition to vitamins, there are nineteen minerals and trace minerals essential to humans and they are grouped into four categories based on their function. Calcium, phosphorus, magnesium, and zinc are structural components of bone. A second group, sodium, potassium, and chloride function as major charged ions within the cellular mechanism. Trace minerals, which are necessary for normal health, include iron, zinc, copper, selenium, manganese, molybdenum, cobalt, iodine, and chromium. Minerals are necessary to prevent deficiency states, and the intake of minerals can be low even in the obese but particularly following surgery for morbid obesity. Calcium is the most abundant mineral in the body and plays a vital role in muscular and cardiac activity. It is also essential in blood clotting and the production of some hormones. Excessive intake of vitamins A and D can give rise to high levels of calcium; low levels are associated with low levels of protein and magnesium. Magnesium is an important mineral within cells, and it is involved in many chemical reactions.

CHAPTER 25
VEGAN AND VEGETARIAN DIETS

Veganism is the practice of abstaining from the use of animal products. An individual who follows the diet or philosophy is known as a vegan. Ethical vegans are known as strict vegetarians and refrain from consuming meat, eggs, dairy products, and any other animal derived substances. An ethical vegan is someone who not only follows a plant-based diet but extends the philosophy into other areas of their lives, opposes the use of animal products for any purpose, and tries to avoid any cruelty and exploitation of all animals, including humans. Another term is environmental veganism, which refers to the avoidance of animal products on the premise that the industrial farming of animals is environmentally damaging and unsustainable.

Well-planned vegan diets are regarded as appropriate for all stages of life by the American Academy of Nutrition and Diabetes, Australian National Health, Medical Research Council, the British Dietetic Association, Dietitians of Canada, and the New Zealand Ministry of Health. The German Society for Nutrition, which is a nonprofit organization and not an official health agency, does not recommend vegan diets for children or adolescents or during pregnancy and breastfeeding. There is inconsistent evidence for vegan and diabetes diets providing a protective effect against the metabolic syndrome, but some evidence suggests that the vegan diet can help with weight loss, especially in the short term. Vegan diets tend to be higher in dietary fiber, magnesium, folic acid, vitamin C, vitamin D, iron, and phytochemicals, and lower in dietary energy, saturated fat, cholesterol, omega-3 fatty acid, vitamin

D, calcium, zinc, and vitamin B12. A poorly planned vegan diet may, therefore, lead to nutritional deficiencies that nullify any beneficial effects and may cause serious health issues, some of which can only be prevented with fortified foods or dietary supplements. Vitamin B12 substitution or supplementation is most important because a deficiency can cause anemia and potentially irreversible neurological damage.

Adopting the vegan diet has become very popular in January and is described as Veganuary. This craze has been described by academics as being potentially unhealthy. That is because those who go on this diet tend to binge on eating meat free junk foods rather than buying fruit and vegetables. They may end up eating meals that are full of salt, fat, additives, and sugar. Vegan burgers and pizzas are often the only options for eating out and are frequently vague and allow snacking on vegan sausage rolls. People can end up eating a less diverse diet including unhealthy vegan meals rather than eating a wider range of foods. Last year 580,000 signed up to the official Veganuary campaign and many more took part unofficially. There is no evidence that plant-based milks such as oat, soya, and almond are any healthier than cow's milk and vegan cheeses are full of carbohydrates. Vegan meals also contain a lot of salt, at least three grams and some over six grams, which is unhealthy.

The American Dietetic Association in 2009 published its position regarding vegetarian and vegan diets, stating they are helpful, nutritionally adequate, and may provide health benefits in the prevention and treatment of certain diseases. Well-planned vegetarian diets are appropriate for individuals during all stages of the lifecycle, including pregnancy, lactation, infancy, childhood, and adolescence, and for athletes. The results of an evidence-based review showed that a vegetarian diet is associated with a lower risk of death from ischemic heart disease. Vegetarians also appear to have lower low density lipoprotein cholesterol levels, lower blood pressure, and lower rates of hypertension and type II diabetes than nonvegetarians. Furthermore, vegetarians tend to have a lower body mass index and lower overall cancer rates.

The Veganuary campaigners have described the following tips for their members. Have a vegan sausage roll or burger no more than once per week. Be aware, meat substitutes often contain harmful chemicals and preservatives. Try to add new vegetables to the diet to get an adequate intake of vitamins and minerals. It is good to make soups containing multiple vegetables. Vegan cheese should be avoided. Additional proteins can be provided from lentils, baked beans, and mushrooms, and many protein drinks are available in supermarkets, some of which contain twenty or thirty grams of protein in a relatively small drink, but they may contain a significant amount of carbohydrates. Vegans should try not to compensate their diet by eating extra sugary snacks. If you need a snack, take mixed nuts and remember that your diet is deficient in vitamin B12, which can be replaced by over-the-counter tablets.

Vegetarianism is the practice of abstaining from the consumption of red meat, poultry, seafood, and the flesh of any other animal, and it may also include abstaining from byproducts of animal slaughter. Vegetarianism may be adopted for various reasons. Many people object to eating meat out of respect for animal life. Some motivations are health-related, political, environmental, cultural, aesthetic, or economic. There are many variations of the vegetarian diet. Some include eggs but not dairy products, while others include dairy products but not eggs.

Western vegetarian diets are high in carotenoids but low in omega-3 fatty acids and vitamin B12. They provide high levels of dietary fiber, folic acid, vitamins C and E and magnesium, and low consumption of saturated fat, all of which are considered to be beneficial aspects of the vegetarian diet. A well-planned vegetarian diet can provide all nutrients in the meat-eating diet to the same level for all stages of life. Protein intake in vegetarian diets tends to be lower than in meat diets but the diets provide sufficient protein intake as long as they contain a variety of plant sources. Iron intake can be maintained but vitamin B12 is not usually present in plants but is abundant in animal products. It can be obtained from dairy products and eggs. Calcium intake in vegetarians and vegans can be similar to that in nonvegetarians provided the diet is properly planned. Broccoli and kale contain calcium that is well absorbed in the body though the calcium content per serving is lower than that contained in a glass of milk.

Meat can be produced in a laboratory and may be more environmentally sustainable than regularly produced meat. Whole cities have been reported to go vegetarian at least once a week, such as

Ghent in Belgium, which introduced a weekly meatless day. The flavors produced by a vegetarian diet can be excellent but public opinion overall maintains a low acceptance rate, which could be changed if the descriptive words focus less on health aspects and more on flavor. Meat is an excellent source of protein but is the most expensive source. Always try to cutoff the fat from the red protein or remove the skin from chicken or turkey. Eating fish is an excellent source of protein, in particular salmon and tuna. Canned fish, however, may be very high in calories but oily fishes are protective against heart disease and are high in omega3 fatty acids. Eggs are a good source of protein and only contain about seventy-five calories and a lot of nutrients, including folic acid, iron, and zinc. Beans are a good source of protein and are low in fat. They also contain a lot of fiber, which is lowest in cholesterol, and reduces the rate of absorption of carbohydrates. Even canned beans are a healthy source of protein nutrition. Nuts contain a lot of fat but mainly monounsaturated and polyunsaturated fats, which are heart healthy. They are rich in vitamin E and fiber. It has been claimed that eating nuts contribute to a prevention of heart disease. Berries supply an excellent source of nutrients, the best probably being blueberries. A cup of blueberries contains a lot of nutrition and fiber while containing less than 100 calories per serving. They are rich in phytochemicals and flavonoids that prevent cancer. It has also been claimed that blueberries improve mental capacity and memory. Olive oil contains monounsaturated fatty acids and antioxidants. It has been claimed to have a role in lowering blood pressure, preventing heart disease, and inhibiting cancer.

GREEN VEGETABLES

Salads have become increasingly popular even in restaurants. Lettuce and tomatoes form the basis for other more exciting foods but can help one to stay inside overall calorie limits. There are several different types of lettuce; the ones that contain most nutrients are arugula, butter lettuce, chicory, and watercress. Tomatoes have a high concentration of antioxidants that are protective against cancer. They may also be instrumental in lowering cholesterol levels.

The ABCs of excellent vegetables are the A's: artichokes, asparagus, aubergenes; B's: blueberries, blackberries; C's: cabbage, cauliflower, and celery. Blueberries contain antiaging properties including better heart health and delayed cognitive aging. They are the best form of nutrition, so add them to your breakfast.

THE GENETICS OF OBESITY

It is usually stated that genetic factors do not play a major role in underlying the basis of the obese state. There are some rare genetic problems that can produce massive obesity, such as Klinefelter's syndrome. A recent study has discovered quirks in DNA that may occur in some obese people, and this could lead to more reliable DNA tests showing someone's risk of developing obesity. Scientists analyzing blood samples from 8809 people in Europe found 202 regions of the genetic code linked to metabolism. They looked at metabolites, the molecules produced when the body breaks down food, alcohol, or medications. Among these, seventy-four were discovered to influence whether a person was obese. These studies could lead to people getting an accurate genetic "risk score" for obesity. The findings are still early but experts hope that a clearer idea of the genetic risk of obesity will emerge from data on half a million people's blood metabolites, which has been made available for study. More research could help to develop drugs to prevent obesity by blocking the genes involved in causing it.

Chapter 26
Dietary Methods for Reducing Weight

The task of losing a large amounts of weight and sustaining the reduction is always major. To lose 100 pounds, which many people need to do, if you try to achieve a negative balance of input over output of energy of 1000 calories per day it would take you thirteen months, and achieving a 1000 calories per day negative balance is not easy it requires a strict adherence to a dietary regime with supplemental exercise and modification of lifestyle. If a person is 100 pounds overweight, he or she is carrying 100 pounds of excess fat and that amounts to 400,000 calories that they need to eliminate.

It has been estimated that, at any one time, two thirds of women and one third of men are trying to lose weight and few of them are successful in the long term. Over one third of the population are regular users of one or more slimming products, most of which are specifically advertised as helping weight loss and are available in the general marketplace. Overall, most attempted slimming is self-administered and self-controlled without supervision. There are, however, no authoritative guidelines for health education in the general public regarding the optimal type of diet.

Over-the-Counter Diets

A wide variety of methods are in use for unsupervised slimming. Many magazines are devoted to the subject and the supermarkets display the slimmest breads and crisps as well as low-energy soft drinks. Over-the-counter items such as meat loaf-based products, which are deemed to reduce hunger by providing bulk to fill the stomach, are widely available. However, there is no scientific evidence that these are of any value in reducing food intake or producing weight loss in the long term. Furthermore, some vegetarian diet dishes bought supermarkets can be very heavy in calories in view of additives containing carbohydrates and fats.

Calorie counted meals are widely available in supermarkets and the recordings of the calorific value of foods in restaurants are becoming more popular, but there is no evidence that they can be relied upon as a vehicle for long-term weight loss. Organizations and magazines run self-help groups. The magazines give substantive advice on slimming, but often perpetuate incorrect nutritional principles. They frequently advocate crash diets, which almost invariably lead to a rebound weight gain, or they focus on specific foodstuffs that may be inappropriate for long-term strategy in achieving weight loss. The most successful of the self-help organizations is Weight Watchers (WW), which is discussed in more detail below.

Historically, diets have focused on reduced fat intake. For over half a century, emphasis has been placed by the medical profession on lowering cholesterol and reducing the intake of animal fat in dairy products. Now the focus has shifted to reducing carbohydrate intake and carbohydrate excesses are converted into fat and are the major problem underlying the obese state. You should let the right foods be your medicine. Eat more green plants, broccoli, cauliflower, asparagus, zucchini, berries, particularly blueberries and nuts, and avoid processed foods. A study in 2019 of 20,000 men and women aged between twenty-one and ninety years found that a diet high in processed foods resulted in an 18 percent increased risk of death from the major killers.

Successful slimming is difficult and clearly depends on the number of factors, many of which are not appreciated subjectively, but the subject's ability to keep to a particular dietary regime is as important as total energy intake. Many individuals find it difficult to sustain any regime for a prolonged period of time, which is necessary, and some diets may be complicated, hard to produce, and expensive.

Calorie Counting Diets

On calorie counting diets, the subject is allowed to eat any foods that cumulatively stay within a given energy intake. Although there is freedom of choice, there are many disadvantages. Food needs to be weighed precisely, and energy intake is calculated from this, but this can be difficult. Commonly, patients will state that these diets fail when, in reality, it is unlikely that the patient has managed to adhere strictly to the dietary requirements. A slight variation on this theme is the set diet, in which a diet sheet provides the week's menu for three meals per day. These menus offer variety and alternatives are frequently given. These are diets such as Nutrisystem, which provide a rich variety of food but in very small portions and by no means the healthiest of foods. Some vegetarian diet meals bought in supermarkets as stated can be very high in calories.

Low Fat Diets

With low fat diets, the individual is provided with a list of foods that are high in fat and must be avoided or severely restricted. These diets often originated specifically to reduce cholesterol levels and thereby reduce the risk of heart disease. Carbohydrates are not usually specifically restricted with these diets which are, therefore, prone to fail.

Low Carbohydrate Diets

Diets that are low in carbohydrates are the key to weight reduction and actually have been available for many years. Dr. Frederick Banting, who discovered insulin over a century ago, devised low carbohydrate diets for treating diabetes. While these have continued to be used, emphasis has only recently been placed on them as a major strategy in weight loss now that it has been realized that carbohydrates are the real enemy. The most widely used low carbohydrate diets are the South Beach Diet, Sugar Busters!, and the Atkins Diet.

The South Beach Diet

The South Beach Diet claims to promote selective carbohydrates and allows low fat. The aim is to teach reliance on the right carbohydrates and the right fats, the good ones, and enable the patient to live quite happily without bad carbohydrates and bad fats. The claim is that between eight and thirteen pounds can be lost in the first two weeks. This is achieved by eating normal size helpings of chicken, turkey, fish, and shellfish. Vegetables are encouraged in the diet, which also includes eggs and nuts. Salads are encouraged using olive oil as a dressing but avoiding other high calorie dressings such as mayonnaise. Three balanced meals a day are allowed, and eating until hunger is satisfied is encouraged. A dessert may be taken after dinner. Bread, rice, potatoes, pasta, and baked goods are completely prohibited, and fruit is restricted in the early days of the diet. Cakes, cookies, ice cream, and sugar are also banned. Some alcohol is allowed but should be restricted to fifteen units per week for men and twelve units per week for women. It is claimed that most of the weight loss in the first few weeks comes off the abdomen so that clothes sizes are influenced early and physical cravings for food usually disappear for as long as the patient adheres to the program. It is claimed that patients eat fewer of the foods that created those urges in the first place, and also fewer foods that cause the body to store excess fat.

After the first two weeks, phase two is entered. Here fruit is allowed, and a small amount of rice or cereal may be introduced. The subject continues on this phase until the ideal weight is achieved. Thereafter, in phase three, the subject is requested permanently to stay on a less restricted form of this diet, and this will ultimately become a way of life in the long term.

It is of interest that the South Beach Diet was devised by Arthur Agatson, a cardiologist who became disillusioned with a low-fat, high carbohydrate diet that the American Heart Association had recommended. As a consequence, he introduced the South Beach Diet in the mid-1990s. Focus was still placed on the prevention of the myriad of heart and vascular problems that stem from the obese state. While placing emphasis on beneficial effects to the cardiovascular system, Dr. Agatson also realizes the importance of the cosmetic effects of losing weight as a strong motivating factor for continuation with the diet. The physiological lift that comes from an improved appearance benefits the entire person and keeps many patients from backsliding. The end result is cardiovascular health with a better, more active, and more positive habitus and attitude. The diet is also aimed at treating the other major killers.

An important principle of the South Beach Diet is to permit good carbohydrates and vegetables. Ultimately, fruits and whole grains may be taken and curtail the bad carbohydrates, the highly processed ones from which all of the fiber has been stripped away during the manufacturing process. To make up for the cut in carbohydrates, the diet permits the intake of fats and animal proteins. The reason for this is that the so-called heart healthy diets were very difficult to stick to because they relied too heavily on the dieter's ability to eat low-fat over a long term. The South Beach Diet encourages lean beef, pork, veal, and lamb provided the fat is removed. This diet also allows eggs, which contain a lot of vitamin D and have a positive effect on the balance between good and bad cholesterol to be taken. Chicken, turkey, fish, especially the oily ones such as salmon, tuna, and mackerel, are recommended, along with nuts, low-fat cheeses, and yogurt. Olive oil, canola oil, and peanut oil are allowed in moderation as these contain good fats. This diet allows some carbohydrates because severe limitation can lead to the breakdown of fats, producing ketosis. To otherwise healthy overweight individuals, this diet is not harmful, but may be associated with a decrease in blood volume and some dehydration, which could in the long term possibly affect kidney function. In a clinical trial including forty overweight volunteers, the South Beach Diet was compared to the American Heart Association low-fat program. After twelve weeks, five patients in the American Heart Association diet had given up, compared with just one on the South Beach plan. South Beach dieters experienced a mean weight loss of 13.6 pounds, almost double the 7.5 pounds lost by the heart Association group. Those on the South Beach Diet also showed a greater decrease in waist to hip ratio, suggesting a true decrease in cardiac risk. Cholesterol levels dramatically decreased for those on the South Beach Diet, and their good-to-bad-cholesterol ratio improved more than that in those on the American Heart Association diet. In addition, much of the insulin resistance syndrome disappeared within the first few weeks on the South Beach Diet. The cravings for sugars and starches were also virtually gone.

After two weeks, fruits and bran or oatmeal are allowed. At this stage, a little whole grain bread can also be introduced into the diet. It should not be spread with jelly but a light covering of butter is allowed. Potatoes are banned. Eggs should be boiled or poached and not fried. Fruits with the lowest glycemic index are strawberries, blueberries, and raspberries, and these are encouraged. Bananas have a high glycemic index and should be avoided; tomato ketchup is not allowed as it is loaded with sugars. Tomato slices, however, are fine. Lettuce, pickles, and onions are perfect. Green peppers, garlic, mushrooms, mustard, and olives are good. Raw broccoli is excellent. Broccoli is covered with a layer of nutritious fiber and the carbohydrate content is slowly absorbed. Not only is the frying of potatoes bad, but even when boiled, the glycemic index remains high as boiling makes the carbohydrate content more suitable for rapid absorption. The digestion of fats and proteins along with carbohydrates, which is allowed, slows the speed with which the carbohydrates are rendered suitable for absorption and, therefore, prevents a rapid rise in blood sugar concentration. A little olive oil will enhance the process of slowing down the absorption of carbohydrate, hence the practice, which is often recommended, of taking a spoonful of Metamucil and a glass of water about fifteen minutes before a meal. Non-soluble fiber mixed with the food has the effect of slowing the speed with which the stomach digests food and also the rate at which the stomach empties is slowed, thus reducing the rate of absorption of carbohydrates.

Word of Warning: the Importance of What We Drink

In many ways, what we drink is more critical than what we eat! The stomach empties liquids more rapidly than solids, rendering them suitable for quick absorption and, therefore, carbohydrate containing liquids have an extremely high glycemic index leading the blood sugar concentrations to rapidly increase. As has been pointed out, there is something of the order of nine or ten teaspoons of sugar in a can of Coke. If pure water is drunk it has the effect of diluting the content of the stomach and slowing down the absorption of solid foods. Therefore, water, as much as you can drink, is recommended.

Beer has a high glycemic index as a result of its maltose content, which makes it even worse than table sugar. Coffee may be protective to the heart and is, therefore, not discouraged, it can however stimulate the stomach to secrete more acid and thereby increase the rate of digestion. A further effect of this is that the increased rate of gastric emptying may increase appetite. Tea also contains caffeine and may also be useful in the prevention of cardiac disease and possibly even prostate cancer. According to the protagonist of the South Beach Diet, wine is less damaging than white bread; it is less fattening.

Outcomes Achieved with the South Beach Diet

It is common for people to lose eight to twelve pounds in weight during the first two weeks of the South beach diet. This is very encouraging for diet participants, but most of the initial weight loss is due to loss of carbohydrate intake, which results in a loss of water storage and water loss from restricting carbohydrate equalizes after about ten to fourteen days. Therefore, thereafter, weight loss slows. A similar result can be achieved by suddenly stopping large amounts of alcohol intake.

Proponents of the South Beach Diet strongly recommend an exercise program, but in moderation, so that the exercise program becomes only a slight intervention in normal lifestyle, rather than a major new discipline. For most people, a brisk twenty-minute daily walk is recommended at least, but can only be expected to burn about 100 calories. The majority of benefit from exercise is gained during the first twenty minutes. Weight training has many benefits. It improves muscle-to-fat ratio, increases metabolism, and promotes the body to burn fuel faster, even when sleeping. Increasing lean body mass, that is body weight from anything other than fat, has a helpful effect on weightlifting. Weight training is also helpful for women in preventing osteoporosis. Furthermore, exercise lowers blood pressure and increases good cholesterol. The developer of the South Beach Diet, Agaston, who is a cardiologist, in addition to adhering to his own diet from promoting further weight loss, takes aspirin and fish oil capsules and uses testosterone gel. Body pump classes are a very good form of exercise; the burning of increased calories can continue for up to six hours after stopping the exercise.

The proponents of South Beach Diet place emphasis on eating patterns. Multiple meals stimulate less overall secretion stimulus to insulin than one or two large feedings. Large feedings are dangerous because they produce a peak of sugar absorption, insulin secretion, and promote insulin resistance. Long periods of fasting alter the body's response to insulin by causing it to enter the conservation mode. The latter tends to cause fat storage. It is, therefore, recommended that people should strive to consume three balanced meals per day with an absence of snacking between each of these, and the longer period between them the more beneficial it will be to retaining good health.

THE SUGAR BUSTERS! DIET

The Sugar Busters! diet emphasizes that sugar is toxic. It is stressed that overproduction of insulin causes the body to store excess sugar as fat, which is insulin resistance. Insulin further inhibits the mobilization of previously stored fat, and insulin signals the liver to make cholesterol, so too much sugar clearly is bad. The Sugar Busters! diet prohibits carbohydrates that cause an intense insulin response. These are the refined sugars. Foods that must be eliminated from the diet are potatoes, corn, white rice, bread from refined flour, beets, carrots, granulated sugar, corn syrup, molasses, honey, sugar colors, and beer. Red wine is allowed with the Sugar Busters! diet. For those who consume alcoholic beverages, the one that is most beneficial appears to be red wine. Populations in countries with a higher relative consumption of red wine to other spirits experienced a lower incidence of cardiovascular disease. Alcohol, however, is high in calories. With the Sugar Busters! diet, as with all diets, exercise is regarded as a definite plus.

Modulating insulin, therefore, is the key underlying the Sugar Busters! diet. Successfully controlling insulin is stated to allow the patient to unlock improved performance through health and nutrition. To control insulin, it is fundamental that the intake of sugar is controlled and that refined carbohydrates are cut down to a minimum. Avoiding refined carbohydrates results in lower average insulin levels in the blood throughout any given period. This has a markedly beneficial effect on reducing fat synthesis and storage as well as mitigating other adverse influences that insulin has on the cardiovascular system. Again, it is emphasized that it is refined carbohydrates that do the damage; unrefined carbohydrates, however, require more digestive breakdown and are, therefore, more slowly absorbed. The slower absorption modulates insulin secretion, reduces peaks in blood sugar concentration, and results in less fat synthesis and storage, so consequently there is less weight gain.

The Sugar Busters! diet does not ban all carbohydrates. There is a particular emphasis on avoiding refined sugars. Many diets advocate eliminating almost all fat and meat, especially red meat. Although many people do not eat too much fat, some fat in the diet is necessary to synthesize steroids, lipoproteins, and other substances necessary for the proper metabolic operations of the body. Ingested fat plays little role in excessive fat accumulation in the body. Most of the excessive fat is due to conversion of ingested carbohydrates to fat. Proponents of the Sugar Busters! diet place great emphasis on the eating of meat. Ingested protein stimulates glucagon secretion as well as providing the building blocks for the body. Glucagon promotes the breakdown of stored fat and helps counteract the effects of high insulin levels on the cardiovascular system.

With the Sugar Busters! diet, alcohol, in reasonable amounts is considered beneficial. Alcohol increases HDL cholesterol and decreases platelet stickiness and aggregation, which can lead to vascular thrombosis. These actions tend to reduce the development of arteriosclerosis and are particularly likely to be achieved when red wine rather than other forms of alcohol is ingested. It has been shown in a number of studies that the number of deaths from cancer, heart disease, strokes, and accidents are cumulatively reduced in people who take one or two alcoholic beverages per day but not more than three. Those who drink more than three run a higher relative risk of death from all causes. The consumption of alcohol remains somewhat controversial, and views are highly conflicting.

The proponents of the Sugar Busters! diet placed emphasis on eating patterns. Multiple meals stimulate less overall insulin secretion than one or two large feedings. Long periods of fasting alter the body's response to insulin by causing it to enter the conservation mode. This tends to increase fat storage. It is, therefore, recommended that we should strive to consume three balanced meals every day. Sugar Busters! expresses concern about eating too much fat, especially saturated fats. With multiple meals per day, portion size is very important. The portions of food selected for each meal should fit on the bottom of the plate and should not extend over the sides. Second and third helpings are actively discouraged. It is beneficial to consume calories early in the day, and the eating of large meals late at night is forbidden. Ingested cholesterol, it is thought, leads to elevations in serum cholesterol and deposition of cholesterol in the arterial system. Between meals, snacks should consist of fruits with the exception of watermelons, pineapples, raisins, and bananas all of which have a high glycemic index. Fruits contain the basic sugar fructose and stimulate approximately one third of the insulin secretion that is created by glucose. Consequently, fruit alone as a snack is beneficial. Taken in combination with other carbohydrates it loses the advantage of lowering insulin secretion that is achieved when eaten by itself. Fruits should be eaten whole and fruit juices are discouraged because they inevitably contain a large amount of sugar. Sugar Busters! recommends consuming fluids between, and particularly, before meals rather than at the time of eating. They discourage the overconsumption of regular coffee and tea as a result of the caffeine stimulus, which can interfere with sleep. Caffeine also makes the stomach secrete more acid, which stimulates appetite and may upset the stomach. Drinking water throughout the day will discourage the desire for food, thereby helping weight control. Breakfast cereals are discouraged. Most breakfast cereals are laced with either white sugar, brown sugar, molasses, corn syrup, or honey. In fact, it is difficult to purchase a pure natural grain cereal. Those based on oats are the healthiest. Wheat bread is allowed in the form of whole grain rather than whole meal.

The Sugar Busters! diet is thus aimed at reducing insulin secretion while enhancing the secretion of glucagon. The ultimate effect is a reduction of body fat and cholesterol as well as the many health problems created by both of these. Adequate sources of protein are a must. Forms of lean meat such as beef, fish, and fowl are recommended. These should have the fat removed and should be grilled, baked, or broiled, since frying involves the use of saturated fats. Other excellent healthy protein sources are eggs and nuts with possibly a little cheese, but not too much of the latter. The proponents of this diet use the aphorism of "lighting the grill and throwing away the frying pan." Sugar Busters! claimed to be creating a new nutritional lifestyle and a new form of healthy individual. It is logical, practical and reasonable. It aims at removing unnecessary fat, especially saturated fat from the diet, and concentrating on the ingestion of lean and trimmed meats. Refined carbohydrates are strictly forbidden, but starches may be taken in moderation. The Sugar Busters! diet is a useful guide to a weight loss program. It is healthy and safe but it does not need to be pursued in the long term once the normal weight range has been achieved, and further advice on one's day-to-day diet will be discussed later.

THE ATKINS DIET

The Atkins Diet was claimed by the late author to be an easy to stay with regime that combines nutrition and vita-nutrient supplements to a unique, weight-reducing, age-defying program. Atkins claimed that this diet added many years to life, boosted the immune defenses, and enhanced brain function and memory. It was also claimed that it reduced the risk of cardiovascular disease and permitted weight loss without calorie restriction, and combated adult onset diabetes. The longer-term assessment of the outcomes of this diet put into question some of Atkins initial premises such as a reduction of cardiovascular disease, which may in fact be increased by the diet. Atkins promulgated his diet against strong opposition from bodies such as the American Heart Association, who themselves have come under criticism with regard to the strategy that they have been promoting for many years.

The Atkins Diet involves a radical reduction of intake of carbohydrates. Those carbohydrates that are allowed are the complex and unrefined ones, basically starchy foods including whole grains and lentils. Table sugar, sweets, cakes, cookies, and soft drinks are banned. These latter foods all have a high glycemic index that sends insulin levels and blood sugar concentrations soaring. Simple carbohydrates should be no more than 3 percent of the total diet. Pasta, bread, white rice, baked goods, candy, and soda are forbidden.

Atkins promotes little restriction on the ingestion of fats. He points out, however, that trans fats are the dietary link to elevated cholesterol and heart disease. Trans fats lower the good HDL cholesterol and raise the bad LDL cholesterol and lipoproteins. Trans fats also reduce responsiveness to insulin and the uptake of essential fatty acids. He also emphasizes the use of safe food products with the avoidance of those animal foods that contain antibiotics or hormones. He advocates the taking of a wide variety of foods that will supply an array of vital nutrients and phytochemicals and avoid any potential of addiction to a particular foodstuff or produce vitamin and mineral deficiencies.

The first objective of the Atkins Diet is to stabilize blood sugar concentrations as is the case with the previous two diets discussed. This again is achieved by eliminating most simple carbohydrates and sugar containing foods and replacing them with other complex carbohydrates or non-carbohydrates.

The diet is based on the much higher than normal fat and protein content and certainly much higher than that which is promoted with the South Beach or Sugar Busters! diet. A second objective of this diet is to create the intake of foods low in oxygen free radicals and high in the antioxidants that fight them. To increase antioxidant capacity, the diet is very high in fresh vegetables and low-sugar fruits such as berries.

An advantage of the diet as with those previously discussed is that the patient does not have to count calories or even excessively restrict portion size. He stated that steak and fish may be eaten with free access to fresh vegetables. Brown rice and whole grain bread is allowed. Some cheeses are permitted, but yogurts, which are high in lactose, a simple sugar, should be kept to a minimum. Bran is allowed and nuts and seeds are encouraged. Atkins recommended taking butter rather than margarine, stating that margarines contain large amounts of trans fats that release cascades of artery-damaging free radicals. Remember that butter and margarine are very high in calories, but fat intake helps to stabilize blood sugar concentrations. Recommended are the monounsaturated vegetable oils such as olive, almond, avocado, and macadamia. These oils are excellent sources of omega-3 and omega-6 fatty acids. The consumption of complex carbohydrates is allowed as these are more likely to maintain the blood sugar at a steady level, particularly when combined with protein and fat. Generous and varied portions of salad greens, broccoli, kale, Brussels sprouts, and green beans are encouraged. Potatoes are again discouraged. Vegetables are better than fruits; the latter should only be taken in moderation. Fruits are a good source of fiber, vitamins, minerals, and other essential nutrients but contain significant amounts of simple carbohydrates and fruit juices, which have added sugars, and are to be avoided. Canned fruits have virtually no nutritional value and are loaded with added sugar and should be avoided. The drinking of tea is allowed, but Atkins discourages coffee consumption. Alcoholic beverages may again be taken in moderation. Beer and dessert wines, however, should be avoided.

Choices among fruits or berries are of any kind but frozen berries frequently have added sugar. A cup of blueberries, which are about the best of all the berries, contains about ten grams of carbohydrates, which is only forty calories. Avocados are an excellent source of monounsaturated fat and are, therefore, healthy fats. It has been stated recently that carotenoids such as lycopene may help to prevent cancer, particularly cancer of the prostate. This has now been added to many of the over-the-counter vitamin preparations. Sources of these are dark green leafy vegetables and carrots, with high concentrations being present in tomatoes.

A disadvantage of the Atkins Diet is that with such a somewhat extreme reduction in carbohydrates the body does not burn fat efficiently and produces compounds called ketones, which accumulate in the blood. These sometimes cause nausea, headache, fatigue, bad breath, and constipation. They can put a strain on the kidneys. There is some debate now as to whether this diet increases the risk of heart disease, vascular disease, and even cancer because of its relatively high concentration of fats. Ironically, perhaps the diet has been shown to be associated with lower levels of serum cholesterol. Overall, the Atkins Diet is now dated and has been superseded by the two previously discussed low carbohydrate diets, both of which are to be preferred over the more extreme Atkins Diet. The question of an increased risk of heart disease remains, which is what Atkins himself died from.

High-Protein Diets

The Eades diet is essentially a low carbohydrate diet that depends upon the rationale of eating large amounts of protein to improve lean body mass but not stimulate insulin, and therefore, the overall effect is a slimmer, healthier body. It is also encouraged for people to eat only a small amount of fat. This is quite probably a good diet for athletes and weightlifters, but it is expensive. High protein drinks such as "Lean Body" contain a large amount of protein up to forty grams in a single drink and relatively small amounts of carbohydrate. These drinks are good.

It has recently been claimed by two Australian academics at the University of Sydney that if you eat too little protein, you will be tormented by cravings and thus likely to overindulge in all the wrong foods. Whereas on a higher protein diet your appetite can be satisfied with fewer calories. It is claimed that if you eat a plate of fish or chicken you won't be tempted to go on eating foods predominant in fat and carbohydrates. The higher protein intake will help us to build muscle and produce enzymes for growth, cell replacement, and repair. We eat too much ultra-processed food lacking in protein, and this results in obesity. These workers claim that eating eggs or fish for breakfast, rather than carbohydrate-laden cereals and bread, hunger and calorie consumption will be reduced later in the day.

It is claimed by the late Dr. Michael Mosley that when hunger strikes you should drink a cup of plain tea or coffee, up to four cups per day. He recommended planning activities or exercise programs to avoid key craving trigger points in the day. We should aim to get 15 to 20 percent of our calories from protein to avoid pangs of hunger. This means eating a minimum of forty-five grams for women and fifty-five grams for men. As you get older you need more protein. A medium-sized egg contains eight grams of protein and provides eighty calories.

Weight Watchers (WW)

A popular diet that has a huge following is the Weight Watchers (WW) diet. This in some ways might seem to fly in the face of the principles outlined above that underlie the strategy for the other popular weight-reducing diets. Whatever the confabulation, I have to say that the Weight Watchers diet is successful for many people and a large amount of weight can be lost by following their principles. This diet has been around for many years and the company has gone through multiple ownerships with many changes. It employs a totally different philosophy strategically based on a point system, and the subject is restricted to staying within a fixed number of points daily. It does not calorie count, as such, and many of the points allocated are perhaps surprising but, again, the system does work.

There are no restrictions on the foods that you can eat, provided that you do not exceed the daily points limit of which there is a maximum and a minimum. Weight Watchers offers as many as 8000 recipes for program participants to choose from. Some foods are surprisingly classed as scoring no points, though obviously, they contain calories. Examples are skinless chicken, turkey breast, fish, and shellfish, and even eggs. Two slices of bread are, however, three points, a Big Mac counts eighteen points, one cup of whole milk is seven points, and a foot-long Subway American club contains thirty-two points. Some of the foods listed as freestyle-no points are the following: apples, beans, broccoli, coleslaw, eggs, mushrooms, onions, salads, and mixed vegetables. You can eat as much of these as you like. Although many aspects of the Weight Watchers diet seem to contradict the principles used in strict calorie-restricted enforcement as stated the system does work and has been beneficial to many thousands, at least in the short term.

It must be said that most diets in the long term ultimately fail. This is largely because people tend gradually to stray away from the restrictions of their diets and, ultimately, while becoming disillusioned, return to their old bad habits.

It has recently been reported that more than 2000 dieters with type II diabetes put on a regime of soup and shakes to reverse diabetes lost on average of thirty pounds in just three months. Previous studies have found that half of people with type II diabetes can reverse the condition if they adhere to strict diets for several months that reduce calories to about 800 a day, provided that they maintain their weight loss in the long term. Further studies are being carried out on over 10,000 people. This study showed good adherence to the diet with intense commitment to the food replacement products for three months, before being put on a plan that reintroduces healthy foods. This study was targeted at those aged between eighteen and sixty-five, with a body mass index of over twenty-seven who had a type II diagnosis for at least six years and were of black, Asian, or minority ethnic origin. These people being those at highest risk for diabetes and its complications.

All of the above diets I have described place emphasis on drinking large amounts of water, at least eight glasses per day, or calorie-free drinks, which in itself is not easy to achieve. Fruits and vegetables contain a large amount of water, but basically all of the essential vitamins and minerals required for good health.

It has long been known that there are groups of people in the world who live extraordinarily long periods of time while maintaining good health throughout their lives. These long-living people are the Abkhazians of Russia, the Vicabanbans of Ecuador, and the Hunzukuts of Pakistan. There is no obesity in these societies, and they all live amazingly disease-free lives. It is also claimed that there is neither cancer nor heart disease amongst them. Their diet is essentially comprised of fruits and vegetables.

I am not trying to advocate that you live your lives firmly attached to any of these diets, which are principally designed to achieve weight loss, but they all in their various ways illustrate what is involved in healthy eating and what foods should be avoided. They are all based on the underlying principle that refined carbohydrates are bad for you and that these are the major cause of all of the diseases killing us in present day society.

Chapter 27
An Exciting New Development That Could Potentially Change the Playing Field

The Daily Telegraph has recently reported that weight loss jabs are as effective as the gastric band and are now going to be prescribed by the NHS in Great Britain. The National Institute of Health and Care Excellence has given the green light to Wegovy, a once weekly injection that suppresses appetite.

Trials have found that those put on the treatment lost an average of almost forty pounds compared with those given a placebo. Researchers have claimed that the treatment is a game changer, with results comparable to those of weight loss surgery. One third of those taking part in a randomized, controlled clinical trial lost an average of one fifth of their total body weight.

The new recommendations are that the treatment should be given to those with a body mass index of thirty or over in particular to those with a body mass index of thirty-five with a weight-related health problem. More than one in four people in the United Kingdom are obese, which means that they have a body mass index of thirty or over. Experts have said that the treatment, which is manufactured by the pharmaceuticals company Novo Nordisk, should be taken alongside changes in dietary habits and exercise habits, the latter of which are fundamentally important.

The drug works by hijacking the body's own appetite regulating system in the brain, leading to reduced hunger and calorie intake. The research found that those put on the regime lost five times as much weight as those in the placebo group. When the results were published, Rachel Batterham, the lead researcher for the project and professor of obesity at University College London said that this was "a major breakthrough for improving the health of people with obesity." "No other drug has come close to producing this level of weight loss—this really is a game changer," she said.

"For the first time people can achieve, through drugs, what was only possible through weight loss surgery." If this holds true, in the long term, it could put into question the whole practice of obesity surgery, which is high risk and often in the long term fails. Britain has some of the worst rates of obesity in the Western world, with as many as two in three adults being overweight or obese. As a retired surgeon who has performed over a thousand gastric bypass procedures for the morbidly obese, I would be delighted if the new drug could replace the need for this surgery, which is major, possibly life threatening, expensive, and tends to fail in the long term. Presumably, the drug treatment could be repeated if necessary.

Chapter 28
Conclusions: How Do I Stay Healthy?

In conclusion therefore:

1. The most damaging foods are those which contain large amounts of low molecular weight carbohydrates. Fats are essential to a healthy diet, the best ones containing large amounts of omega-3 and omega six fatty acids. Proteins are the most healthy form of calories but red meats are not as healthy as white meat so it is best, largely, to base your diet on the eating of chicken, turkey, fish and green vegetables.

2. We can best control calorie intake by adhering to the above recommendations that will provide an adequate nutritional and vitamin content. The best diet to follow in my opinion is the South Beach diet but I would not discount the use of Weight Watchers, which while not as scientifically based it does have a number of positive effects which are well documented.

3. I have underlined the basic principles of nutrition with an emphasis on eating protein and essential fats but minimizing the intake of low molecular weight carbohydrates. A healthy diet should provide an adequate intake of vitamins and essential mineral nutrients, but an additional multivitamin preparation can be helpful provided that the dose is not exceeded.

4. In participating in the taking of a good diet it should be emphasized that nutrition affects the mind, and the most appropriate diet is capable of increasing intellectual functioning.

5. Forms of energy that are most healthy are good proteins, essential fats with concentrations of Omega three and Omega six fatty acids and large molecular weight carbohydrates such as those found in green vegetables.

6. Providing essential energy intake is best achieved by adhering to a healthy balanced diet as indicated above.

7. For the morbidly obese person, that is those with a body mass index in excess of 40, the best solution has been to undergo surgical treatment, but with the advent of the semaglutide drugs, such as Wegovy and Ozempic, it is possible that these may be a forerunner of, or even replace surgery. If surgery is chosen the best operation for the morbidly obese is the Roux-en-Y gastric bypass, amounting to a loss of up to 60 or 70% of extra weight in 18 months, many are unable to sustain this degree of weight loss and ultimately after 18 months there tends to be weight gain. There is no place for the Lap Band, the results of which have been very disappointing. Therefore, the risk of weight gain without adequate disciplinary control of calorific intake is considerable.

8. Exercise programs are an important part of attaining overall a healthy body. They promote the ability to participate in healthy exercise, tend to reduce the effects of aging, and, from a psychological point of view, are excellent. They cannot, however, be regarded as a major fundamental strategy in achieving significant weight loss for the obese. The obese also may find exercise programs difficult to participate in both, because of the difficulty in achieving what is required in the program and the psychological factors that may prevent them from joining a group in the gym and entering an exercise program therein.

9. Emotional stress is for many a major factor in producing a negative overall health outcome. It predisposes to depression, lack of healthy social contacts and failure to adequately participate in a healthy social contact group. Failure to adequately participate in

a healthy eating program as a result of having undergone excess weight gain is a common ultimate outcome. It is important to try to avoid anxiety by visualizing outcomes and not dwelling on past negative experiences, the latter of which can increase and cause excessive worrying later in life. If possible, try to avoid anger, fear, sadness and frustration. Think positively.

10. With regard to optimizing vitamin and mineral intake, the balanced diet should be adequate but taking a single multivitamin preparation, of which there are many, each day can be recommended.

11. Achieving a healthy sleep pattern which amounts to approximately seven hours sleep per night can be a major factor in both promoting physical and mental health in the long term. This can be achieved by organizing one's lifestyle along the above recommended lines and avoiding late evening consumption of a heavy meal or a large amount of alcohol.

12. With regard to alcohol consumption, up to two glasses of red wine per day may contribute to good health. Otherwise, the amounts recommended for an adult are a weekly intake that should not exceed 20 units for a male and 16 units for a female.

13. You should try to get an annual physical examination with a full blood count, chemical and thyroid, and also measurement of vitamins D, B, iron and magnesium.

14. With regard to life extension, Jeff Bezos, Elon musk, and Bill Gates are investing in a new anti-aging company, Altos Labs, which is going to look at cellular DNA and its modifications in order to extend life. This is attempted by turning adult cells into embryonic stem cells that have the capacity to repair and replace damaged tissue. This may help to make people's elderly years healthier rather than extending life per se. It has now been shown that the taking of a healthy diet can protect telomere caps on the ends of strings of chromosomes, that protect genes by replication, this is thought to have the potential of extending life in the long-term.

Today some of the finest scientific minds are dedicated to exploring the genes and cells in our body to enable us to cope with the aging process and keep us healthier for longer. "Rejuvenation science" is now a big business in Silicon Valley. New ideas are hitting the track such as injecting the elderly with a young person's blood. Bizarre as this may seem it could possibly work. Older mice injected with the blood of younger mice saw a boosting in the proteins responsible for repairing damaged tissue as well as better brain, muscle, and liver function. This treatment is being funded by the US Government's National Institute for Health.

The quest for immortality is no longer the focus, as this largely depends upon one's genes. It is now about extending the period of healthy life expectancy or "health span." The key aim is to narrow the gap outlined at the beginning of this book, that is a twenty-seven-year difference in life expectancy between different geographical areas in the UK. In the seaside town of Blackpool healthy life expectancy stands at fifty-five years compared with seventy-one years in the wealthier areas of Southeast England. Experts are trying to find ways of keeping people healthier longer, to reduce the period of loss of active function at the end of lives.

What is the strategy? Well, one idea is to give healthy people medicines that treat diseases such as cancer and diabetes years before they actually develop the disease.

One drug on which the emphasis of the research has been based in the USA relates to the use of an antibiotic rapamycin, which is usually given to organ transplant patients. In dogs this drug has been shown to improve cardiac function in the elderly and prevent heart problems later in life. This resulted in an increase of 38 percent in preserved energy later in the animal's life. Human studies at Stanford University have shown that older people given a six-week course of rapamycin had and unusually strong antibody response to the flu jab an developed fewer infections compared to a matched group who were not given the drug.

Currently there are more than 2000 trials looking at the antiaging effect of rapamycin. Another widely used drug being investigated is the diabetes treatment drug metformin, which has been used since the 1950s to reduce blood sugar levels. Studies have found, coincidentally, that people who take this drug live longer than those taking other diabetes medications and even longer than those who don't have diabetes. The drug is thought to produce the same effect as fasting or reduced calorie intakes, which have a well-proven antiaging benefit. Calorie restriction has been shown to have a rejuvenating effect on damaged cells. The lack of nutrients causes the body to break down its own cells for energy, and the first to get used are those that are damaged or malfunctioning. This causes a culling of old, half dead cells, which could have gone on to cull the killing diseases later in life, while a greater proportion of healthy cells remain. Fasting causes the body to start using fat stores for fuel, which stimulates the release of a chemical shown to promote new connections in the brain, possibly boosting cognitive function. Rapamycin and metformin are thought to have the same effect. Another drug, dasatinib, has been shown to increase lifespan by 25 percent in animals and to improve heart and kidney function later in life. These new drugs possibly also protect the retina and improve eyesight.

Finally, one can say with an increasing degree of scientific certainty that the major killers of people in the Western World are due primarily to identifiable DIETARY FACTORS and the optimal conditions for a healthy lifestyle, which I would recommend, are most principally related to a healthy diet and the abandonment of smoking. It can be said that damage incurred can be a reversible entity, so it is never too late to change one's eating habits. In addition, taking an adequate amount of exercise per day and sleeping well with as much avoidance of stress as possible are important factors.

An outline of these factors is briefly illustrated below in ten points, as a guideline to establishing a healthy daily dietary regime.

1. After getting up in the morning, drink a cup of coffee with skimmed milk.
2. Take a walk sometime in the morning for about half an hour approaching 5000 steps.
3. Have breakfast, ideally consisting of a boiled egg, blueberries and Kiwis, and a single slice of whole meal toast buttered. Drink as much water as you can throughout the day.

4. Try to avoid midmorning snacks, drink water or calorie-free drinks if hungry.
5. Have a light lunch, preferably a green salad.
6. In the evening, take a second walk and trying to achieve another 5000 steps, walking the dog is good.
7. Before 9 PM eat the main meal of the day, preferably white meat, turkey, or better still fish, say salmon. Add mixed vegetables, cheese, asparagus, broccoli, cabbage, cauliflower, peppers, onions or shallots and add olive oil. Have one or at the most two glasses of wine, preferably red, and restrict desserts to twice a week.
8. Rest, watch television, listen to the radio, or play music later in the evening.
9. Go to bed before 11 PM, make sure that the bedroom is dark, don't watch television in bed, though you can read and then hopefully get seven to eight hours of uninterrupted sleep.
10. Try to avoid the issues, throughout the day, that make you anxious.

Even with this relatively disciplined approach the evening meal can be very palatable, exciting and nutritious. Let me give you one example for your home cooking.

Chicken Spaghetti Casserole

Prep time 25 minutes

Cook time 35 minutes

Total time : 1 hour

Servings: 6 servings

Calories: Less than 300

Source modified from recipegirl.com. Weight Watchers Main course

Cuisine: American

INGREDIENTS

- 7 ounces thin spaghetti
- 1 tablespoon of salted butter
- 2 cups of sliced mushrooms
- 1 onion, chopped
- 1/2 cup of chopped celery
- 1/2 cup of chopped green bell peppers
- Two 10.75-ounce cans 98 percent fat free cream of mushroom soup
- 1 cup of skimmed milk
- 4 ounces of reduced fat cheddar cheese
- 2 cups of chopped cooked chicken breast
- 1 teaspoon of Tabasco sauce
- Pepper and a little salt, to taste
- 1/2 cup of shredded Monterey Jack cheese

PREPARATION

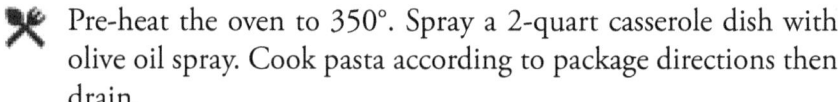 Pre-heat the oven to 350°. Spray a 2-quart casserole dish with olive oil spray. Cook pasta according to package directions then drain.

Melt butter in a large skillet over medium heat. Add mushrooms, and bell peppers celery. Cook until the vegetables have softened, four to five minutes.

In a medium bowl, mix milk and soup. Add this to the vegetables in the pan. Add a sprinkling of cheese and continue to heat until it has melted, and the sauce is smooth. Add in chicken, pasta and some tabasco sauce.

Pour the mixture into a casserole dish and sprinkle the jack cheese and bake for 35 minutes, or until the casserole is hot and bubbly.

You have a delicious main course in little over an hour for less than calories. It contains 29 grams of protein, 30 grams of carbohydrate, an grams of fat. Rich in vitamins and minerals—enjoy it, it is delicious and healthy.

Chapter 29
Established Diagnostic Eating Disorders

Anorexia Nervosa, Bulimia and Food Cravings or Addiction

Anorexia nervosa has been well recognized for over 50 years and its prevalence has increased and continues to increase yearly, but little is known of the underlying cause which remains elusive and nothing has been recently added to its treatment. This is a condition in which a major underlying factor is a fear of being fat and it can develop from an early age. The onset of anorexia nervosa most frequently occurs during the teenage years. The vast majority of cases are females but the number in males is also increasing. The condition has the highest mortality rate among all the psychiatric disorders. The eating disorder takes control of the individual and is their primary focus in life. Sufferers focus on the specifics of extreme calorie intake and food avoidance together with excessive exercising, usually walking which is all they have the strength to do.

The description of anorexia nervosa as a mental illness remains controversial but it is not uncommonly associated with other recognized mental diseases such as depression. Little is known about the factors which originate the anorexic problem, various theories exist which are widely disputed. Patients can deteriorate until they live on the brink of death, and they often influence their family and others in a deleterious way. Bulimia nervosa, in which subjects repeatedly induce post prandial vomiting, is associated with anorexia in some cases. The patient develops a distorted body image when they think they are fat though in reality they are marasmic. They restrict and avoid food intake though the bulimics may binge eat and vomit. Not all bulimics are underweight some are slightly overweight but they still suffer from physical and mental damage. The subject may become secretive, evasive, and dishonest, frequently hiding and destroying food as they are desperate to avoid gaining weight. Someone may have told them that they look fat or they themselves feel that they are obese. Sometimes it may be a reflection of their mother being fat. There is an association in some with sexual abuse at an early age. The patient's social life becomes nonexistent, particularly as there is animosity around any food and they feel that they do not look good, so they become increasingly isolated. They rarely seek advice though friends and relatives frequently call their attention to the situation. The fear of being fat, however, overwhelms any tendency to be honest or integral and the compulsions the disease creates can continue and progress for many years. Treatment frequently fails and multiple body organs can be damaged, sometimes permanently. Muscle wasting and weakness is common leading to profound fatigue and difficulty in performing day-to-day functions. Orthostatic hypotension which produces a feeling of weakness and unsteadiness with instability on standing from the sitting position is common and precipitated by an underlying low blood pressure and poor venous return to the heart. Calcium deficiency leads to osteomalacia and osteoporosis, thinning and weakening of the bone predisposing to fractures following minor trauma. Hormone imbalance is frequent causing loss of the menstrual cycle and painful bone, and joint disease is frequently witnessed such as coccydynia, severe pain at the lower end of the spine on sitting down. A common manifestation is the development of lanugo, the presence of soft, fine down or white hair on the face, back and forearms. This is thought to be a response to hypersensitivity to cold and is thought to be protective.

Mood swings and depression are common, often influenced by dehydration and electrolyte disturbance, hormone and vitamin deficiencies. Anorexia is frequently associated with symptoms of obsessive-compulsive disorder. There may be a family history of depression. Intellectual disturbances can also occur but frequently the subjects of anorexia are highly intelligent though introspective.

The disease can have wide impacts causing family problems, problems in the workplace and they can be damaged by bullying when bullies detect their bodily damage and subsequent weakness.

Prolonged fasting may damage the liver and is a major cause of liver failure in young people, chronic heart failure which develops also adversely affects liver function. Alcohol intake or abuse is rare in the anorexic. Lowered body temperature and malnutrition can cause heart arrhythmias and heart failure. vitamin and mineral deficiencies develop vitamins A and C, iron and iodine deficiencies occur and are associated with respiratory infections, kidney failure, visual disturbance and ultimately death. Electrolyte disturbances can cause cardiac arrhythmias and even cardiac arrest. Low potassium levels can arrest the heart causing cardiac muscular damage or even cardiac arrest, the blood pressure falls causing orthostatic hypotension and a slow heart rate. Neuromuscular disorders can occur as a result of vitamin and mineral deficiencies. Iron deficiency anemia frequently develops impairing oxygen carriage to the tissues and causing breathlessness, weakness, infections and heart arrhythmias. Kidney failure is exacerbated by a combination of hypotension, electrolyte disturbances, protein deficiency and urinary tract infections. Edema can result from low protein concentrations in the blood and the use of laxatives and diuretics.

Esophageal reflux is common particularly in the bulimic and this can lead to damage to the lining of the esophagus and to produce Barrett's esophagus which can lead to esophageal cancer. Vomiting in the bulimic can cause a tear in the lining of the lower esophagus, the so-called Mallory Weiss syndrome. The fingers can become calloused by repeated vomiting resulting from putting them down the throat to induce it. The vomiting can also damage tooth enamel and dental problems are frequent even sometimes resulting from scurvy.

Enhanced understanding in this area could be a crucial step in disrupting the dominant cultural constrictions underlying eating disorders. When health and management of illnesses are considered as personal moral responsibilities people with body forms coded as different or abnormal have increasingly become the objects of media exposure which can be damaging, particularly as the nature of the underlying disorders are not fundamentally understood. Individuals with eating disorders resist the critical labels identifying them. This can make the anorexic uncooperative or even hostile, thus exacerbating the problem. The media present slim attractive women who are successful as a state to be strived for and the process of weight loss in achieving this may lead to anorexia which will then accelerate and go beyond this goal leading to a disorientated view of their own body image and an intense fear of reversal to an overweight state.

The patient who is severely affected by anorexia requires hospitalization and reversal of their malnutrition. This requires isolation, frequently intravenous nutrition, and in extreme situations disconnection of wash basins in the room so that vomiting can be detected. Following discharge from hospital relapse is very common and ultimately the only possibility of reversing the inexorable damage is dependent upon the patient voluntarily reversing the situation and many can ultimately get back to a normal lifestyle and maintain a normal weight.

Binge eating disorders occur when a much larger amount of food than normal is taken in a short time. Binging can be a factor in the bulimic but also occurs intermittently. What sets binge eating disorder apart from others is the lack of purging and the high frequency of binging, two or more times weekly.

The triggers to binge eating are extremely mood sensitive, susceptible to hormonal changes, fatigue, life events, or disappointments with oneself or with others. Vulnerable sufferers may feel a binge coming on and gather food in advance, or may just eat whatever is at hand, even food they don't ordinarily like. Bingers usually eat alone, at home, to hide the amount or the types of food consumed, but they also begin at a party or restaurant when a normal amount is eaten but the overeating continues at home. The key feature is, once started, the Binger feels out of control, compelled to keep eating to the point of discomfort and even misery. Subsequently the Binger feels ashamed and disgusted, but unable to stop doing it again and again. This leads to a chronic feeling of guilt and dread of discovery—thus addictive behavior.

Food cravings have a continuously disruptive effect on attempts to diet and constitute a continuous goad to binge eating behavior. Researchers have been teasing out the difference between craving, needing, and liking certain foods, independent of hunger. Virtually 100 percent of young women and 70 percent of young men have experienced food cravings during the past year. Contrary to popular opinion, a craving is not in response to a body deficit of nutrients or calories. Food cravings, alcohol, and drug cravings all use the same brain pathways. The image of food or drugs invokes more intense reactions than the substance itself. This suggests the powerful role of habit which is reinforcing these biologically bound food cravings. The same pattern of increased craving is clearly demonstrated when a person attempts to stop smoking, another area where habits and cravings strongly overlap. Even after stopping, the former smoker may experience cravings when presented with any smoking related situation or memory. So too, certain life situations may bring on a food craving. Antidepressants and mood stabilizing medications may be useful in aiding mood regulation and dealing with craving and compulsive eating.

Anorexia Nervosa Treatment

Anorexia nervosa is a psychological disorder resulting from an intense fear of fatness and weight gain. It is associated with a distortion of body image. The mortality from the condition is about 1 percent; 80 percent of these die from the effects of marasmus and 20 percent from suicide. The disease has the highest mortality rate of all mental disorders. The condition is difficult to treat, associated disorders such as depression and anxiety frequently complicate treatment.

Treatment involves primarily improving the nutritional state with protein adequate calorie intake and sometimes the addition of essential vitamins and minerals. A fundamental disorder of the thinking process needs to be addressed as soon as possible, and low self-esteem needs counseling.

Patients with anorexia nervosa are sensitive and secretive about their problem and are frequently opposed to undergoing treatment. The disease can go on for many years and the longer, the worse is the outcome. Treatment begins with consulting the general practitioner and frequently seeing a clinical psychologist. Frequently psychiatric treatment is required but there is no established form of drug therapy. Associated disorders, depression, anxiety, self-harm, obsessional symptoms and suicide attempts need special therapy.

Attempts must be made to get the patient's weight up to the normal range and to establish a normal eating pattern which may be difficult and is frequently resisted. Severe cases require inpatient hospital treatment in a single room and parenteral (intravenous) feeding may be necessary.

The mainstay of treatment in the longer-term case is cognitive behavioral therapy which guides the patient to a realistic view of the situation and attempts to establish an understanding of the magnitude of their problem. It is a personalized clinical intervention specifically designed to proactively address all of the difficulties encountered.

CHAPTER 30
IN CONCLUSION

Most of the major killers of people today were rare a century ago, although clearly the overall dynamics of the lifecycle in Western society have dramatically changed. We have, however, inherited a new constellation of killing disorders that are almost uniformly causing our deaths, and these have a single unifying course, which wasn't a factor a century ago, and that is diet—bad diet. We have eaten our way into the predominant deadly diseases like coronary artery disease, heart failure, diabetes, hypertension, stroke, most forms of cancer, and Alzheimer's disease by bad diet. Most of these are potentially avoidable with a relatively easy-to-achieve change in our dietary habits. The major culprit is the massive consumption of refined carbohydrates 150 times the amount eaten a century ago compared with 1g. The ingestion of proteins is good, and fats can no longer principally be regarded as the major cause of early death. Simple sugars are the enemy.

The world population is now 7.8 billion. Eleven percent are in Europe and 5 percent in North America; 83 percent can read, 75 percent have mobile phones, 30 percent have Internet access, but only 7 percent have a university education. Currently, two thirds of the worldwide population died between the ages of fifteen and sixty-four, and only 8 percent live to be sixty-five or over. If you are over sixty-five, you belong to a very select group. You need to be careful and extending your longevity depends on eating the right diet.

Please remember that it is fundamentally not about living longer. It is about having a healthier life throughout old age without disabling and life-threatening comorbidities. These latter manifestly disable people at about the age of sixty, leaving them with perhaps twenty years of compromised lifestyle ahead. It is never too late to begin with dietary modification and exercise. Start right away by modifying your diet along the lines described above. Walk, cycle, or swim, and perhaps join the gym. It could reverse your ills, making you more productive and less dependent in later life. The exciting new group of drugs, the semaglutides, Ozempic, Wegovy and others have been reported to achieve the same amount of weight loss as weight-reducing surgery, could completely change the playing field for the better and overcome the pandemic of destructive eating in the most vulnerable group of people. As a surgeon who has previously carried out over one thousand gastric bypass operations, I would welcome the development of a drug that could rival surgery in its results and possibly eliminate the need for surgery, which is major, potentially dangerous, expensive, and often fails in the long term, whereas the medication could potentially be repeated if weight regain occurred.

1. Which foods are damaging?

   Perhaps now, ironically, refined carbohydrates are the most damaging foods which are the primary contributors to diabetes, arteriosclerosis, heart disease and stroke.

2. How can we control calorie intake?

   Controlling calorie intake is the essence of maintaining a healthy weight. The best way to curtail excess calorie intake is to eat meals predominantly consisting of white meats, fish and as many green vegetables as you like. There can obviously be some flexibility and to make life more interesting you can deviate from this but not excessively. You should avoid too many cakes, cookies, pies and other sweets.

3. What are the basic principles of nutrition?

   The basic principles of nutrition are that in order to maintain good health we need to eat a good balance of energy giving foods of which there are three basic constituents, carbohydrates, fats and proteins. Proteins are the healthiest, we need these for muscle and growth, fats are essential, the healthiest are Omega three and Omega six fatty acids, the worst are the saturated fats. We need carbohydrates for energy and for brain health, but too much refined carbohydrate is really bad, large molecular weight carbohydrates found in vegetables are the best. Containing total energy consumption in terms of calorific count is of fundamental importance. Eating a balanced diet, without excessive calorie intake, is essential in providing necessary vitamins and minerals without this recognized deficiency diseases develop.

4. What are the major sources of energy required for nutritionally a healthy body?

   Energy comes from three basic sources, carbohydrate and protein provide four calories per gram, fat contains 9 cal per gram. You should try to get most of your nutrition from protein, fat and large molecular weight carbohydrates found in vegetables and reduce the amount of refined carbohydrates such as those found in sweets, cakes and cookies.

5. What to do about vitamins and minerals?

    A well-balanced diet will provide all the essential vitamins and minerals which you need. There are eight essential vitamins and 13 major essential minerals of which the most prevalent in the body is calcium. Many multivitamin products are available in all pharmacies and taking one of these tablets a day as a dietary supplement is acceptable.

6. How do we need to convert energy intake along with eating healthily?

    Eating a healthy diet containing 2000 cal per day for men and 1600 cal for women will provide adequate energy.

7. What is the most healthy and economically viable weight reducing diet?

    In my opinion the best weight reducing diet, which is economically viable and well tolerated, is the South Beach Diet. Mediterranean diets have also been shown to be very healthy?

8. What should we do about optimizing exercise?

    Taking adequate exercise is a very important component in maintaining a healthy body. It will help you to diet but in itself will produce only a little weight loss. Walking burns about 350 cal per hour, cycling 450 cal per hour and running or swimming up to 600 cal per hour. Perhaps paradoxically running a marathon will burn about 3500 cal which is less than the number consumed in a Thanksgiving dinner. The amount of exercise taken varies with age, clearly most premier league football players retire from the game in their mid-30s, for the elderly the best forms of exercise are walking and swimming. In addition, going to the gymnasium can be excellent particularly when performing exercises such as body pump.

9. How important is stress and its control in the equation?

    Stress and depression can often lead to weight gain and are bad for us in so many ways.

10. Are there any medications which we could use prophylactically?

    Absolutely, and this may represent the most major breakthrough in the treatment of the obese state and all its complications for all time. A new group of drugs the semaglutides, the most well-known of which are Ozempic and Wegovy, have been shown in clinical trials to produce appetite suppression and marked weight loss, the use of these drugs may ultimately challenge the need for bariatric surgery. The demand for this group of drugs is now huge but there are some side effects, mainly related to gastrointestinal upsets.

11. How much time should we spend sleeping?

    Ideally, we should spend about seven hours per night sleeping.

12. How much alcohol is it safe to drink?

    The amount of alcohol which is safe is controversial. 14 units per week for a man and 12 for a woman is probably safe and may even be beneficial. Much excess of this and particularly binge drinking is dangerous, possibly leading to cirrhosis and liver failure. It has been maintained that Red-wine is good and a glass of red wine only contains about the same number of calories as a slice of bread. It may be that red wine in moderation can be preventative in coronary artery disease.

SUGGESTIONS FOR FURTHER READING:

Overcoming Obesity. Thomas Taylor, Vantage Press.

Working With Weight. Thomas Taylor, Stratton Publishing.

Lifestyle and Longevity. Thomas Taylor, SBPRA.

Upper Digestive Surgery. Thomas Taylor et al, Saunders Amazon.

Prediabetes for Dummies. Rubin, A L, Wiley.

The Mayo Clinic Diabetes Diet. Amazon.

Vaccinology, Morrow et al, Wiley.

The Science of Sleep. Heather Darwell, Smith.

This is Your Brain on Food. Uma Naidoo, Amazon.

Eat Drink, and Be Healthy: The Harvard Medical School Guide to Healthy Eating, Amazon.

We'd like to know if you enjoyed the book. Please consider leaving a review on the platform from which you purchased the book.

www.ingramcontent.com/pod-product-compliance
Lightning Source LLC
Chambersburg PA
CBHW052031030426
42337CB00027B/4949